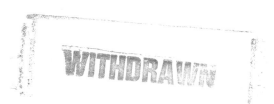

PREVENTING & MANAGING
OSTEOPOROSIS

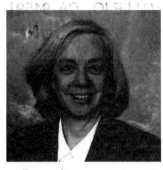

Sarah Hall Gueldner, DSN, is Professor and Director of the School of Nursing at The Pennsylvania. State University, with a dual appointment in the College of Medicine. She also holds an affiliate faculty appointment and serves on the Advisory Board for Penn State's Gerontology Center.

Dr. Gueldner earned a Bachelor of Science in Nursing degree from the University of Tennessee College of Nursing in Memphis, a Master of Nursing degree from Emory University, and a Doctor of Science in Nursing degree from the University of Alabama in Birmingham, where she was named Medical Center Graduate Fellow. She completed postdoctoral study in psychoneuroimmunology at Emory University. Dr. Gueldner held an appointment as a Senior Research Scientist at the University of Georgia Gerontology Center from 1988–1994 and is a Fellow in the American Academy of Nursing and the Association of Gerontology in Higher Education.

Her research program centers on health promotion in elderly populations, with secondary work related to instrument development. She served as the Principal Investigator for a federally funded study that examined the benefits of exercise in nursing home residents and community-dwelling elders, and has completed studies focusing on exercise, environmental enrichment, expression of mood, life satisfaction, and immunocompetence in elderly populations.

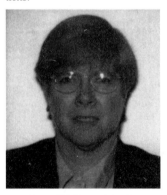

M. Susan Burke, MD, FACP, is a native of Philadelphia. She is a graduate of Chestnut Hill College in Philadelphia, where she received a B.S. in Biology in 1975. She attended the University of Pennsylvania School of Medicine where she graduated in 1979, and subsequently completed her residency in Internal Medicine at the Lankenau Hospital in 1982. Dr. Burke has been the director of the Lankenau Hospital Medical Clinic; she also serves as preceptor for medical students of Thomas Jefferson University, where she is Clinical Assistant Professor of Medicine.

In 1992, Dr. Burke was the recipient of the Osler-Blockley Award from Jefferson University for excellence in teaching medicine at the bedside, and in 1993 was elected Fellow of the American College of Physicians. The Residents' Award for Best Teacher was awarded to her in June 1997 by the Lankenau Internal Medicine housestaff. Dr. Burke is board certified in Internal Medicine and Geriatrics, and lectures nationally on numerous geriatric topics including osteoporosis, osteoarthritis, and cardiovascular disease.

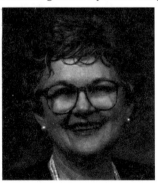

Helen Smiciklas-Wright, PhD, is Professor of Nutrition and Director of the Diet Assessment Center in the Department of Nutrition, The Pennsylvania State University. She received her B.S. and M.S. degrees from the University of Toronto and her Ph.D. degree in nutrition from The Pennsylvania State University. Her research interests are in assessment of older adults who are at nutritional risk and the antecedents and consequences of risk. Current projects include a longitudinal study of rural older adults and food-medicine safety study. Dr. Smiciklas-Wright and her colleagues are currently initiating intervention studies in collaboration with the Geisinger Regional Health Care System.

PREVENTING & MANAGING
OSTEOPOROSIS

Edited by

SARAH HALL GUELDNER, D.S.N.
M. SUSAN BURKE, M.D., F.A.C.P.
HELEN SMICIKLAS-WRIGHT, PH.D.

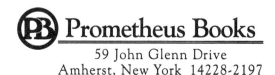
Prometheus Books
59 John Glenn Drive
Amherst, New York 14228-2197

Published 2003 by Prometheus Books

Inquiries should be addressed to
Prometheus Books
59 John Glenn Drive
Amherst, New York 14228–2197
VOICE: 716–691–0133, ext. 207; FAX: 716–564–2711
WWW.PROMETHEUSBOOKS.COM

07 06 05 04 03   5 4 3 2 1

Library of Congress Cataloging-in-Publication Data

Preventing and managing osteoporosis / edited by Sarah Hall Gueldner, M. Susan Burke, and
    Helen Smiciklas-Wright.
        p. cm.
    Previously published: New York : Springer Pub., 2000.
    Includes bibliographical references and index.
    ISBN 1–59102–027–1 (alk. paper)
    1. Osteoporosis. I. Gueldner, Sarah Hall. II. Burke, M. Susan. III. Wright, Helen S.,
1936–
RC931.O73 P73 2002
616.7'16—dc21

                                                                            2002031844

Printed in the United States of America on acid-free paper

Contents

Acknowledgments

Preventing and Managing Osteoporosis is an outgrowth of Stand Tall, Pennsylvania, an educational project sponsored by the Geriatric Education Center of Pennsylvania (GEC PA), a consortium of the Gerontology Centers at The Pennsylvania State University, the University of Pittsburgh, and Temple University. This project involved the collaboration of many individuals, and the editors are indebted to each of them.

We especially acknowledge the enthusiastic support of K. Warner Schaie, PhD, GEC PA Co-Director; and Susan B. Keller-Hoover, MPH, GEC PA Project Coordinator, both of Penn State University. Other key leaders of the consortium lending energy to this effort include Richard Schulz, PhD, GEC PA Director, University of Pittsburgh; Albert J. Finestone, MD, GEC PA Co-Director, Temple University; John G. Hennon, EdD, GEC PA Associate Director, University of Pittsburgh; Kathleen A. Segrist, PhD, GEC PA Project Coordinator, Temple University; and Diane Ives, GEC PA Research Assistant, University of Pittsburgh. Our thanks also to Melvin Horwith, MD, College of Medicine, Penn State University, for helping us to build the network of expertise needed for the completion of this book.

We would also extend our sincere appreciation to Ursula Springer and the editors and staff at Springer Publishing Company for their interest in this important topic and for their skillful guidance in bringing this book to print. Credit also goes to Merck Laboratories and the National Osteoporosis Risk Assessment Project for sharing materials they developed for inclusion in this book.

In addition, the editors would like to take this opportunity to thank Janice Penrod, Gail Shirk, and Cindy Musser for their extensive editorial assistance; and Anna Lombard, Janette Moore, Jean Barczak, Leah Salter, Susan Cherry, Pamela Reed, and Kathie Conklin for the technical assistance necessary for the completion of this book.

Foreword

Osteoporosis is a disease process that from late midlife on can have devastating effects on the successful aging of most women and many men. The consequences of adverse changes in posture and increased risk for severe damage, which often occur during falls when bone density has been significantly reduced, are not only physical in nature, but often result in a serious reduction in life quality and the ability to function independently in the community. Hence, the need to understand osteoporosis and its consequences goes beyond seeing the process as a medical treatment issue but addresses as well the psychosocial factors involved in its prevention and management.

This book provides a useful introduction and overview of the disease process, its epidemiology, interventions to prevent this condition, and ways to manage osteoporosis when it does occur. It will be of use to clinicians in virtually all health-related disciplines, including physicians; nurses; nutritionists; psychologists; gerontologists; exercise physiologists; occupational, physical, and recreational therapists; as well as adult day care and long-term-care directors. The book is written in an accessible manner so that it will also be a useful resource for persons suffering from, or at risk for having, osteoporosis and those individuals who serve as informal caregivers for these persons.

This volume is one of the outcomes of a curriculum development project that was designed to raise the awareness and increase knowledge in various groups of health professionals in relation to the prevention, early detection, and management of osteoporosis. The project was sponsored by the Geriatric Education Center of Pennsylvania (GEC), which is a consortium effort conducted by the Gerontology Centers at The Pennsylvania State University, the University of Pittsburgh, and Temple University, with grant support from the Health Services and Resources Administration. Credit also goes to the Penn State site coordinator of the GEC, Susan Keller, who took on a leadership role in assembling the research faculty and practitioners who developed the curriculum model, most of whom are represented in this volume. Ms. Keller also took a leading role in assembling the curriculum model and in field testing it with a professional audience.

K. WARNER SCHAIE, PhD
Evan Pugh Professor of Human Development and Psychology
Director, Penn State Gerontology Center

Contributors

Jane A. Cauley, DrPH
University of Pittsburgh
Graduate School of Public Health
Department of Epidemiology
130 Desoto Street
Pittsburgh, PA 15261

Ellen Field-Munves, MD
Springhouse Professional Center
1575 Pond Road
Suite 202
Allentown, PA 18104

Philip Hanus, PharmD, BCPS
Director, Pharmaceutical Care
Penn State Geisinger Health System
100 North Academy Avenue
Danville, PA 17822

Eric D. Newman, MD
Director, Department of
    Rheumatology
Penn State Geisinger Medical Center
100 North Academy Avenue
Danville, PA 17822

Roberta Newton, PhD
Department of Physical Therapy
Temple University
3307 North Broad Street
Philadelphia, PA 19140

Janice Penrod, MS, PhD(C)
    (Candidate)
Research Assistant
School of Nursing
201 Health and Human Development
    East
The Pennsylvania State University
University Park, PA 16802

Susan Rankin, PhD
Senior Diversity Planning Analyst
Office of the Vice Provost for
    Educational Equity
313 Grange Building
The Pennsylvania State University
University Park, PA 16802

K. Warner Schaie, PhD
Evan Pugh Professor of Human
    Development and Psychology
Director, Gerontology Center
Human Development and Family
    Studies
105 Henderson Building South
The Pennsylvania State University
University Park, PA 16802

Delores C. Schoen, PhD, RNC,
    FAAN
Adjunct Faculty
School of Nursing
The Pennsylvania State University
229 Horizon Drive
State College, PA 16801

Gail B. Shirk, MS, CRNP
Nurse Practitioner
Vascular Risk Intervention Clinic
Department of Cardiology
MC 21-60
100 North Academy Avenue
Danville, PA 17822

Randi L. Wolfe, PhD
University of Pittsburgh
Graduate School of Public Health
Department of Epidemiology
130 Desoto Street
Pittsburgh, PA 15261

Catherine E. Wright, BS
Science Writing Consultant
229 N. Craig Street, #503
Pittsburgh, PA 15213

1

Introduction and Overview

Sarah Hall Gueldner

> Osteoporosis is a pediatric disease with geriatric consequences.
>
> —M. Drugay

The purpose of this book is to raise awareness and inform front-line health and health-related professionals from across disciplines about the silent but crippling and deadly epidemic of osteoporosis that has been too long dismissed as a normal part of aging. Compelling statistics of the incidence and devastating consequences are included to profile the personal, social, and financial impact of this now preventable and treatable disease. Personal portraits give face and voice to those who must live their last years bent and fragile from bones that give away suddenly and painfully, usually more than once, to the ravages of osteoporosis. Finally, encouraging information is given about recent diagnostic and treatment breakthroughs that enhance our ability to prevent and detect osteoporosis and to better manage its unwelcome sequelae.

Written by a team of authors from medicine, nursing, nutrition, exercise physiology, physical therapy, and demography, the book is intended to be a handbook for clinicians and educators in all health-related disciplines. It also is offered as a quick reference to teachers and other key community figures from all walks of life who are in a position to identify and refer persons at risk for osteoporosis. It is hoped that the book will also be useful to persons who have or are at risk for having osteoporosis, and to their unheralded but gallant informal caregivers. Finally, we would be pleased if every woman who has osteoporosis were to read portions of the book and help us carry the very personal message to their daughters and granddaughters. For they are the most targeted population if we are to rid our towns and communities of the ravages of osteoporosis, as our predecessors spared modern society from polio, small pox, and rickets.

OVERVIEW

The incidence of osteoporosis is occurring at an epidemic level, particularly among postmenopausal Caucasian women, but also in a number of other risk groups, including elderly men and persons of any age or gender who take corticosteroids or anticonvulsants over an extended period of time.

Osteoporosis is defined as "a systemic skeletal disease characterized by low bone mass and microarchitectural deterioration of bone tissue, with a consequent increase in bone fragility and susceptibility to fracture" (Anonymous, 1991). Osteopenia refers to a decrease in bone mass below normal but not severe enough to be classified as osteoporosis.

Osteoporosis is more common in women than heart attack, stroke, and breast cancer combined (Anonymous, 1991). Insidious loss of height and incidence of nontraumatic fractures are the two most prominent clinical presentations of osteoporosis. Until recently, nontraumatic fractures were the telltale signal that almost always announced its presence. The most common sites of such fractures are hips, wrists, and the vertebral bodies of the spinal column.

The specific etiology of the disease remains unknown, but current research has focused primarily on a defect in the normal bone remodeling process and pharmacologic interventions that are designed to modulate this abnormality. A number of encouraging diagnostic procedures and strategies for the prevention and treatment of osteoporosis have become available during recent years, but both health care providers and patients have been slow to acknowledge and use even the most simple and least expensive of these management advances.

Two types of osteoporosis have been identified: primary and secondary. Primary osteoporosis is the type usually referred to as postmenopausal, and secondary osteoporosis refers to the type that is caused by other identifiable disorders, such as (a) endocrine disorders; (b) prescribed drugs or toxic chemicals such as corticosteroids (the most serious offender), heparin, anticonvulsants, immunosuppressants, alcohol, and smoking; (c) chronic diseases such as renal conditions and gastrointestinal disorders that result in malabsorption of calcium and other nutrients; (d) extended debility or immobilization; (e) deficiency states in nutrients necessary for building bone, including calcium and vitamin D; and (f) inborn errors of metabolism.

The characteristic physical changes associated with osteoporosis alter appearance and are generally irreversible. The most obvious deformity, kyphosis ("dowager's hump"), cannot be hidden and worsens over time, eventually affecting other body structures and functions. These conspicuous alterations of physical appearance threaten self-image and may limit the person's range of movement and lead to decreased interaction with other people.

It has been said that of all the undesirable effects of osteoporosis, pain may have the most profound impact on the lives of the individuals it affects. Unfortunately, however, the possibility of pain is not even mentioned in most plans of care. What is perhaps most troubling is the chronicity of the pain; it is a daily burden to bear, with little hope of relief.

As pain and limitation of activity increase, feelings of sadness, hopelessness, and depression are not uncommon. Likewise, the individual with a hip fracture or multiple vertebral fractures becomes increasingly vulnerable to limitations in social activities, which may lead to social isolation. For these reasons, the successful management of established osteoporosis depends on recognition and treatment of its psychosocial and functional components, as well as the improvement of the bone disorder.

In summary, osteoporosis is a complex disease process, intruding on multiple arenas of life in older women and men. No single professional has the time or expertise to manage all of its consequences. The fruits of our research on osteoporosis are finally yielding the diagnostic and treatment options to eliminate osteoporosis in future generations. However, society in general, including its health-related professionals, seems mired in puzzling complacency, unable to embrace the exciting potential to rid civilization of the crippling plague of osteoporosis. The following chapters will attempt to translate the emerging information in a way that will inform and mobilize the entire world community toward this realistic goal.

REFERENCES

Anonymous. (1991). Consensus Development Conference: Prophylaxis and treatment of osteoporosis. *American Journal of Medicine, 90*(1), 107–110.

Drugay, M. (1997). Breaking the silence: A health promotion approach to osteoporosis. *Journal of Gerontological Nursing, 23*(6), 36–43.

2

Epidemiology: The Magnitude of Concern

Randi L. Wolf, Janice Penrod, and Jane A. Cauley

> The silent epidemic of osteoporosis has been challenged.
> We are now beginning to appreciate the magnitude of this
> disorder in our world populations.
>
> —R. L. Wolf

From an epidemiological perspective, definitions matter, because the estimated number of people with osteoporosis depends on how osteoporosis is defined. The 1993 Consensus Development Conference defined osteoporosis as a disease characterized by low bone mass and structural deterioration of bone tissue leading to bone fragility and an increased susceptibility to fractures (Anonymous, 1993). Note that this definition requires both a reduction in bone mass *and* a reduction in bone quality. However, since practical measures of fragility caused by structural deterioration are currently unavailable, we must rely on measures of bone mineral density (BMD) alone. BMD is measured noninvasively where the amount of bone mineral is counted for a given area of bone—usually a section of the hip or spine. The lower the BMD, the higher the risk of fracture and the higher the incentive to intervene with treatment. In fact, prospective studies indicate that for each one standard deviation fall in BMD, the risk of osteoporotic fractures doubles (Cummings & Black, 1995).

Using BMD to assess risk of fracture is similar to using blood pressure to identify those at risk of stroke or using cholesterol levels to identify those at risk of coronary artery disease. By creating categories of BMD, the population at risk of developing osteoporosis or at risk of fracture due to osteoporosis can be estimated. This method of determining the prevalence of osteoporosis was suggested in 1994 by an expert panel of the World Health Organization (WHO).

PREVALENCE OF OSTEOPOROSIS

The World Health Organization has proposed a classification system for women based on BMD measures (Kanis, 1994). A woman's actual BMD is assessed and then compared to the average "peak" BMD of a healthy young adult female reference group. The woman's deviation from this average (statistical mean) is then calculated in standardized units (i.e., standard deviations or SD). So essentially, this system calculates the difference in a woman's current bone density from a referenced peak bone density. The difference is expressed as the number of standardized units (i.e., SD) above or below the average peak density (i.e., the mean).

Based on the WHO definitions, *normal* is used to classify women whose BMD is less than 1 SD below the mean. Those whose BMD is from 1 to 2.5 SD below the mean are classified as having *osteopenia*. Osteopenia, or low bone mass, refers to cases in which the bone loss is not severe enough to warrant classification as osteoporosis. In order to be classified as *osteoporosis*, the BMD must be greater than 2.5 SD below the mean. *Severe or established osteoporosis* is used to describe those who meet this criteria for osteoporosis *and* have a history of fragility fractures. A more detailed discussion of the WHO system of classification is provided in chapter 7.

Using the WHO criteria for osteopenia and osteoporosis, Looker, Orwoll, Johnston, et al. (1997) recently reported the prevalence of low femoral bone density in a sample of 14,646 U.S. men and women who participated in the Third National Health and Nutrition Examination Survey (NHANES III). The reference population was 382 white men and 409 white women, 20 to 29 years of age. According to the WHO criteria, osteoporosis under age 50 was rare. However, 13% to 18% of women aged 50 or older had osteoporosis, and another 37% to 50% had osteopenia. Applying the most recent U.S. census data, this translates to 4 to 6 million women with osteoporosis and 13 to 17 million with low bone mass (osteopenia).

Prevalence Varies by Race and Ethnic Group

Prevalence of osteoporosis in the United States is higher among non-Hispanic white women (13% to 18%) than among Mexican Americans (10% to 12%) or non-Hispanic black women (5% to 8%) of the same age (Looker et al., 1997). But don't be mislead by population-level percentages—even small percentages represent a substantial number of women.

Prevalence Varies by Gender

One percent to 4% of men aged 50 years and older present a BMD warranting classification as osteoporotic, confirming that osteoporosis permeates the lives of about 280,000—1 million men (Looker et al., 1997). Add to that number the 15% to 33% of men with osteopenia (low bone mass), and another four to nine million men enter the picture. These estimates challenge the long-held myth that osteoporosis is a sex-segregated problem.

Prevalence Varies by Geographic Location

Within the United States, the prevalence of osteoporosis varies rather dramatically among the states. States with the greatest number of women and men with osteoporosis include California (14%), Florida (14%), New York (14%), Pennsylvania (14%), and Texas (13%) (National Osteoporosis Foundation, 1997). It is not coincidence that these states also rank highly in proportion of older adult residents.

It should be pointed out that this classification system, though commonly used, has some limitations for estimating prevalence across diverse populations. The applicability of the WHO criteria to groups other than Caucasian women is not certain. Current recommendations are to use a white female reference population for *all* groups (Radiological Device FDA Panel Meeting, 1999), although the appropriate cut-off values for osteoporosis and osteopenia in men and other racial and ethnic groups are still under investigation. In addition, the prevalence of osteoporosis may be underestimated when only a single BMD site (e.g., hip) is used since an individual with normal BMD at one site may have low BMD at another site (e.g., spine, wrist). The prevalence of osteoporosis is expected to be higher if a number of skeletal sites are assessed simultaneously (Melton, Atkinson, O'Connor, O'Fallon, & Riggs, 1998). The limitations are important when trying to determine prevalence rates of osteoporosis in a given population.

FRACTURE INCIDENCE

Of the 1.3 million fractures that occur in the United States each year, 70% of all fractures among individuals age 45 years and older are attributable to osteoporosis (Iskrant & Smith, 1969). Although the disease can affect any bone in the body, the most typical sites of fractures related to osteoporosis are the hip, spine (called vertebral fractures), and wrist (often called Colles' fractures).

When considering fracture rates by age categories, the type of fracture shifts. During one's 50's, wrist fractures are most common. Into the 60's, the most common fracture site shifts to the vertebrae of the spine; and by the 70's, hip fracture becomes the most common site of osteoporotic fracture (Cooper, Campion, & Melton, 1992). The rate of all three types of fracture increases with age, but the increased risk with aging is most pronounced for hip fractures (Melton, 1996).

Lifetime Fracture Risks

Beginning at age 50, Caucasian women have about a 40% chance of fracturing their hip, spine, or wrist in their remaining lifetime (Melton, Chrischilles, Cooper, Lane, & Riggs, 1992). Considered specifically, these women have about an 18% chance of breaking their hip, a 16% chance of vertebral fracture, and a 16% chance of breaking a wrist. Stop to consider the significance of this finding: After age 50, *4 out of every 10 women* face a significant fracture risk, and *one out of every six women* over age 50 faces the risk of hip fracture in their lifetime! This risk is equal to the *combined* risk of developing breast, uterine, *and* ovarian cancer in the remaining years of life.

For men, the estimated lifetime fracture risk is about 13% after age 50 (Melton et al., 1992). The site-specific fracture risks are 6% for the hip, 4% for the spine, and 3% for the wrist. Thus, men have a lower overall rate of fracture than women, but we must not be deceived by seemingly low population-level percentages.

For African Americans, data is available only for the hip. Estimates for lifetime risk are 5.6% and 2.8% for women and men, respectively (Cummings, Black, & Rubin, 1989). These estimates will need to be refined as life expectancy continues to increase and fracture incidence changes over time (Oden et al., 1998).

CONSEQUENCES OF OSTEOPOROSIS

The epidemiological story of osteoporosis would be incomplete without considering the toll of this disorder on public health. Three major consequences pose impact: mortality, morbidity, and cost.

Mortality

Hip fracture is a significant perturbation in health status and poses an increased risk of mortality (death). Mortality with hip fracture is often related to coexisting diseases (or co-morbidities) such as stroke or chronic lung diseases (Browner, Pressman, Nevitt, & Cummings, 1996), or to complications that arise secondary to medical/surgical treatment of the fracture.

Excess mortality occurring after a hip fracture, compared with that expected in the population, is estimated to range from 12% to 35%. A person's age, race (Jacobsen et al., 1992), gender (Jacobson et al., 1992; Ismail et al., 1998; Center, Nguyen, Schneider, Sambrook, & Eisman, 1999), health, and functional status (Browner et al., 1996; Magaziner et al., 1997) contribute to the survival outcome following hip fractures. The greatest excess mortality typically occurs within the first year (Jacobsen et al., 1992); however, some studies show a sustained effect (Magaziner et al., 1997). In one recent report, the greatest excess mortality was within the first six months following a fracture in those with the poorest health; however, there was a continuing trend of increased mortality, with an excess of 14 deaths per 100 cases by five years, for patients who had little functional impairment and few co-morbidities before the fracture (Magaziner et al., 1997). Men appear to have a poorer prognosis than women (Center et al., 1999). A large prospective study showed men had poorer survival outcomes than women for hip, vertebra, and other major (e.g., pelvic, rib) and minor (e.g., distal arm and leg) fractures (Center et al., 1999). In general, African Americans fare relatively worse than their Caucasian counterparts (Jacobsen et al., 1992) in terms of mortality following hip fracture.

Morbidity

Morbidity, the term used to denote living with sustained effects of a health disturbance, is of great concern for persons who suffer a fracture. For most of these people, the effects of the event are sustained. In cases of hip fracture, 40% do not regain their prefracture walking status within a year. More than 50% never recover their prefracture ability to perform physical activities of daily living such as eating, dressing, grooming, or bathing (Magaziner, Simonsick, Kashner, Hebel, & Kenzora, 1990). One study showed that more than half of the men who suffer a hip fracture are discharged to a nursing home and that 79% of these men who survive at one year will reside in nursing homes or intermediate care facilities (Poor, Atkinson, Lewallen, O'Fallon, & Melton, 1995).

In a recent study of a fairly healthy population sustaining a new hip fracture and then discharged to their own homes, gait and balance were assessed two months after the fracture and then patients were followed for the next 2 years (Fox et al., 1998). Both poor balance and poor gait were associated with more admissions to nursing homes (20% and 17% increased odds, respectively). Poor balance, but not gait, resulted in more hospitalizations and increased mortality rates (17% increase with each unit decrease in balance score) following the fracture. Another recent study found that after adjustments for possible confounders, including co-morbid conditions, women with hip fractures were significantly more likely to report difficulty performing 11 out of 15 different tasks, including mobility tasks (e.g., walking two or three blocks), higher functioning tasks (e.g., light housework, preparing meals), and basic self-care tasks (e.g., bathing, dressing) (Hochberg et al., 1998). Thus, hip fracture presents long-term negative effects for those who survive the initial threat to health.

Turning to vertebral fractures, morbidity is a profound concern. Osteoporotic fractures of the spine result in an unnatural pronounced curvature of the spine (called kyphosis) and a loss of height. These fractures are often called crushing fractures—a term that captures the collapse of the vertebral column onto itself. As the spine loses structural support, the rib cage lowers. In some, the rib cage eventually comes to rest on the iliac crests (the bony protrusions above the hips, near the waistline). This downward shift of the body's structural support (i.e., the skeleton) pushes internal organs down toward the abdomen. As a result, people with osteoporosis often present abdominal protuberance (commonly called a "potbelly") as the organs are pressed downward and forward from the thorax.

These structural changes produce concomitant morbidity: height loss, back pain, abdominal fullness, and inhibited breathing patterns. Nevitt et al. (1998) recently reported results from a large prospective study of 7,223 older white women that had spine X-rays at baseline and at a follow-up examination an average of 3.7 years later as part of their participation in the Study of Osteoporotic Fractures (SOF). Compared to women without a spine fracture at baseline, those with at least one new vertebral fracture were more likely to have increased back pain and back disability. Among women who already had a fracture at baseline, those with a new incident fracture had substantial increases in back pain and functional limitations as well.

Many of these problems subsequently affect other health patterns. For example, kyphosis is associated with diminished function, especially mobility tasks like walking and climbing stairs (Ryan & Fried, 1997). Abdominal fullness is often related to early satiety (a term referring to early satisfaction and fullness upon eating) which over time may result in weight loss. Kyphotic changes in posture lead to more shallow breathing, which may have implications should the person require surgery or anesthesia. Over time, severe kyphosis may even lead to chronic lung disease.

The impact of vertebral deformities may be worse for men than for women (Burger et al., 1997; Matthis, Weber, O'Neill, & Raspe, 1998). One recent large study of 15,570 European men and women showed that the associations between vertebral deformities and negative health outcomes (presence and intensity of back pain, functional capacity, and overall subjective health) were stronger in men than women (Matthis et al., 1998). Similarly, in another prospective study conducted in Rotterdam, the Netherlands, stronger associations were found between severe deformities and detrimental health outcomes in men than in women (Burger et al., 1997).

Even wrist fracture poses morbidity concerns. Colles' fractures can result in long-term inability to perform household tasks or personal hygiene. Though the impact on function tends to be underestimated, these fractures may have lasting effects on everyday life.

From a psychological perspective, postfracture morbidity poses a threat to overall quality of life. Several factors discussed above contribute to perceived losses in functional, social, and psychological well-being. For example, limited mobility and functional capabilities, pain, and loss of independence are often direct effects of fracture. Deformity, produced as osteoporosis that invades the spine, is difficult for many to accept. Fear of falling and of subsequent fractures may heighten concerns. Such morbidities

can not be underattended as we consider the toll of osteoporosis on public health.

Morbidities also tend to have a ripple-like effect. They are not limited
to the individual but ripple into the family system. Loss of independence
induces new family roles and responsibilities. Chronic care, offered infor-
mally within the family and coordinated with formal caregivers, has its own
set of demands and burdens that extend into the network of family and
community and ultimately into society at large. Human and monetary costs
of treatment and rehabilitation following fracture are often shared among
family members and are partially assumed by public providers. This disease
reaches into the lives and pockets of us all.

Costs

Monetary costs associated with osteoporotic fractures are astonishing. About
$38 million are spent *per day* to treat these fractures. This daily cost adds
up to about $13.8 *billion* per year (Ray, Chan, & Thamer, 1997). Since
most of these fractures occur among older adults who are no longer employed,
these figures are not heavily weighted by loss of wages. Rather, the costs
are associated with direct care services: inpatient care (62%), nursing home
care (28%), and outpatient service (10%). Hip fractures account for about
63% of these costs, while other sites consume the remaining 37% (Ray et
al., 1997).

Even the group least susceptible to fracture, non-White men, required
$174 million in osteoporosis care in 1995. The significant contribution of
nonhip fractures in men and non-Whites to health care expenditures should
dispel any lingering misconceptions that the impact of osteoporosis is limited
to hip fractures among older White women.

FUTURE PROJECTIONS

Global graying has become a commonplace reality—the population is living
longer, and the proportion of old people within the population is growing.
The fastest growing segment of the population is the oldest-old (i.e., those
age 85 years or more). Consider the ramifications of these demographic
trends on the incidence of osteoporosis and fracture (both highly associated
with increasing age).

Global demographic changes are expected to increase the incidence of hip fracture nearly four-fold by the year 2050 (Cooper et al., 1992). That equates to a growth from 1.66 million fractures (worldwide) in 1990 to *6.26 million* fractures in 2050. The most significant increase in hip fracture rates is expected to occur in third world countries, particularly in Asia. Currently, Asia accounts for approximately 30% of global hip fractures. By 2050, they are expected to account for more than 50% of all hip fractures (Ellfors, 1998).

Interestingly, a recent long-term study over a 65-year period in Rochester, Minnesota, shows that hip fracture incidence rates in both women and men may now be declining. The reasons for this unexpected trend are unknown. However, the population in the U.S. is aging with enough speed that the actual number of hip fractures is speculated to increase in our part of the world (Melton, 1996). Therefore, even if the incidence is declining, an exponential increase in the number of hip fractures worldwide is projected because of these demographic shifts.

Stop for a moment to consider the collective impact of these fractures on the individual, the family, their community, and society. It is a phenomenal concern that demands our utmost attention if we are to avert this trend. Osteoporosis presents a major public health concern. Arresting this disorder should be a major focus of our preventive efforts in the coming century.

REFERENCES

Anonymous. (1993). NIH Consensus Development Conference: Diagnosis, prophylaxis, and treatment of osteoporosis. *American Journal of Medicine, 94,* 646–650.

Browner, W. S., Pressman, A. R., Nevitt, M. C., & Cummings, S. R. (1996). Mortality following fractures in older women: The study of osteoporotic fractures. *Archives of Internal Medicine, 156,* 1521–1525.

Burger, H., Van Daele, P. L., Grashuis, K., Hofman, A., Grobbee, D. E., Schutte, H. E., Birkenhager, J. C., & Pols, H. A. (1997). Vertebral deformities and functional impairment in men and women. *Journal of Bone and Mineral Research, 12,* 152–157.

Center, J. R., Nguyen, T. V., Schneider, D., Sambrook, P. N., & Eisman, J. A. (1999). Mortality after all major types of osteoporotic fracture in men and women: An observational study. *Lancet, 353,* 878–882.

Cooper, C., Campion, G., & Melton, L. J. III. (1992). Hip fractures in the elderly: A worldwide projection. *Osteoporosis International, 2,* 285–289.

Cummings, S. R., & Black, D. M. (1995). Bone mass measurements and risk of fracture in Caucasian women: A review of findings from prospective studies. *American Journal of Medicine, 98,* 245–248.

Cummings, S. R., Black, D. M., & Rubin, S. M. (1989). Lifetime risks of hip, Colles', or vertebral fracture and coronary heart disease among white postmenopausal women. *Archives of Internal Medicine, 149,* 2445–2448.

Ellfors, L. (1998). Are osteoporotic fractures due to osteoporosis? Impacts of a frailty pandemic in an aging world. *Aging: Clinical and Experimental Research, 10,* 191–204.

Fox, K. M., Hawkes, W. G., Hebel, J. R., Felsenthal, G., Clark, M., Zimmerman, S. I., Kenzora, J. E., & Magaziner, J. (1998). Mobility after hip fracture predicts health outcome. *Journal of the American Geriatrics Society, 46,* 169–173.

Hochberg, M. C., Williamson, J., Skinner, E. A., Guralnik, J., Kasper, J. D., & Fried, L. P. (1998). The prevalence and impact of self-reported hip fracture in elderly community-dwelling women: The Women's Health and Aging Study. *Osteoporosis International, 8,* 385–389.

Iskrant, A. P., & Smith, R. W. (1969). Osteoporosis in women 45 years and over related to subsequent fractures. *Public Health Reports, 84,* 33–38.

Ismail, A. A., O'Neill, T. W., Cooper, C., Finn, J. D., Bhalla, A. K., Cannata, J. B., Delmas, P., Falch, J. A., Felsch, B., Hoszowski, K., Johnell, O., Diaz-Lopez, J. B., Lopez Vaz, A., Marchand, F., Raspe, H., Reid, D. M., Todd, C., Weber, K., Woolf, A., Reeve, J., & Silman, A. J. (1998). Mortality associated with vertebral deformity in men and women: Results from the European Prospective Osteoporosis Study (EPOS). *Osteoporosis International, 8,* 291–297.

Jacobsen, S. J., Goldberg, J., Miles, T. P., Brody, J. A., Stiers, W., & Rimm, A. A. (1990). Hip fracture incidence among the old and very old: A population-based study of 745,435 cases. *American Journal of Public Health, 80,* 871–873.

Jacobsen, S. J., Goldberg, J., Miles, T. P., Brody, J. A., Stiers, W., & Rimm, A. A. (1992). Race and sex differences in mortality following fracture of the hip. *American Journal of Public Health, 82,* 1147–1150.

Kanis, J. A. (1994). Osteoporosis and its consequences. In R. Marcus (Ed.), *Osteoporosis* (pp. 1–20). Cambridge, MA: Blackwell Science.

Looker, A. C., Orwoll, E. S., Johnston, C. C. Jr., Lindsay, R. L., Wahner, H. W., Dunn, W. L., Calvo, M. S., Harris, T. B., & Heyse, S. P. (1997). Prevalence of low femoral bone density in older US adults from NHANES III. *Journal of Bone and Mineral Research, 12,* 1761–1768.

Magaziner, J., Lydick, E., Hawkes, W., Fox, K. M., Zimmerman, S. I., Epstein, R. S., & Hebel, J. R. (1997). Excess mortality attributable to hip fracture in white women aged 70 years and older. *American Journal of Public Health, 87,* 1630–1636.

Magaziner, J., Simonsick, E. M., Kashner, M., Hebel, J. R., & Kenzora, J. E. (1990). Predictors of functional recovery one year following hospital discharge for hip fracture: A prospective study. *Journal of Gerontology, Medical Sciences, 45,* M101–M107.

Matthis, C., Weber, U., O'Neill, T. W., & Raspe, H. (1998). Health impact associated with vertebral deformities: Results from the European Vertebral Osteoporosis Study (EVOS). *Osteoporosis International, 8,* 364–372.

Melton, L. J. III. (1996). Epidemiology of hip fractures: Implications of the exponential increase with age. *Bone, 18,* 121S–125S.

Melton, L. J. III, Atkinson, E. J., & Madhok, R. (1996). Downturn in hip fracture incidence. *Public Health Reports, 111,* 146–151.

Melton, L. J. III, Atkinson, E. J., O'Connor, M. K., O'Fallon, W. M., & Riggs, B. L. (1998). Bone density and fracture risk in men. *Journal of Bone and Mineral Research, 13,* 1915–1923.

Melton, L. J. III, Chrischilles, E. A., Cooper, C., Lane, A. W., & Riggs, B. L. (1992). Perspective: How many women have osteoporosis? *Journal of Bone and Mineral Research, 7,* 1005–1010.

National Osteoporosis Foundation. (1997). 1996 & 2015 Osteoporosis prevalence figures: State by state report. Washington, DC: Author.

Nevitt, M. C., Ettinger, B., Black, D. M., Stone, K., Jamal, S. A., Ensrud, K., Segal, M., Genant, H. K., & Cummings, S. R. (1998). The association of radiographically detected vertebral fractures with back pain and function: A prospective study. *Annals of Internal Medicine, 128,* 793–800.

Oden, A., Dawson, A., Dere, W., Johnell, O., Jonsson, B., & Kanis, J. A. (1998). Lifetime risk of hip fractures is underestimated. *Osteoporosis International, 8,* 599–603.

Poor, G., Atkinson, E. J., Lewallen, D. G., O'Fallon, W. M., & Melton, L. J. III. (1995). Age-related hip fractures in men: Clinical spectrum and short-term outcomes. *Osteoporosis International, 5,* 419–426.

Radiological Devices Panel Meeting Summary, May 17, 1999. *www.fda.gov/cdrh/rdp.html.*

Ray, N. F., Chan, J. K., & Thamer, M. (1997). Medical expenditures for the treatment of osteoporotic fractures in the US in 1995: Report from the National Osteoporosis Foundation. *Journal of Bone and Mineral Research, 12,* 24–35.

Ryan, S. D., & Fried, L. P. (1997). The impact of kyphosis on daily functioning. *Journal of the American Geriatrics Society, 45,* 1479–1486.

WHO Study Group. (1994). *Assessment of fracture risk and its application to screening for postmenopausal osteoporosis.* (WHO Technical Report series: 843). Geneva: WHO.

3

Living with Osteoporosis: The Personal Experience

Janice Penrod

> I shudder when I catch sight of my walking profile reflected in a store window.
>
> —P. Horner

Osteoporosis is literally defined as "porous bone." This definition captures the essence of the abnormality—eroded bone tissue is not adequately replaced, and the excavated sites form porous pockets. These pockets destroy the structural integrity of the bone and bone strength is weakened. But what does this microdeterioration mean in terms of living a "normal" life? How do these changes in the bones affect the everyday lives of individuals with osteoporosis?

This query raises an almost automatic answer: the threat of fracture. Fractures certainly pose dramatic changes in how one manages his/her daily life. Epidemiological rates confirm that fracture looms as the most significant threat faced by persons living with osteoporosis—the fallacy is in thinking that fracture poses only short-term changes in everyday life during the acute phase of recovery.

In reality, fractures pose significant long-term changes in the lives of those with osteoporosis. For many, life is irrevocably changed after the incidence of even one fracture. For example, of those who survive a hip fracture, 40% do not recover their premorbid walking ability and over half (51.5%) do not recover their premorbid abilities to perform activities of daily living (Magaziner, Simonsick, Kashner, Hebel, & Kenzora, 1990). Mortality rates are equally astounding. Vertebral fractures are estimated to increase mortality rates by 4%, whereas hip fractures increase mortality by 10% to 20% (Cooper, Campion, & Melton, 1992; Melton, Ilstrup, Riggs, & Beckenbaurg, 1982).

LIVING WITH OSTEOPOROSIS: WHAT WE SEE

Still, even these figures fail to fully capture the human toll of osteoporosis. Behind these statistics are the changed faces of people living with osteoporosis. In the absence of traumatic fracture, the most common presenting feature of osteoporosis is dramatic loss of height. At the root of this phenomenon are vertebral fractures. These fractures are described as "crushing," the vertebrae essentially collapse or wedge, producing classic changes in posture and loss of height. This postural change is termed kyphosis, meaning that the natural curvature of the spine is altered, causing a rounded hump to form in the upper back and noticeable protrusion of the abdomen. This structural collapse of multiple vertebrae lowers the rib cage until it finally comes to rest on iliac crests, causing the abdomen to protrude in a "potbelly." The tilt of the pelvis forces the knees to bend and the stance to widen. In order to hold the head in an upright position, the chin must jut forward, described as "like a chicken—leading head first."

Living with osteoporosis is not like living with high blood pressure or diabetes. Rather, deformity changes outward appearance into the classic clinical picture of osteoporosis. Individuals are "marked" quite obviously by the stamp of this debilitating condition. These physical changes are commonly accompanied by discomfort and eventually by pain. The detrimental effects of such postural changes extend across multiple systems, producing symptoms such as early satiety, constipation, poor lung function, and gait and balance changes.

Viewed within a professional perspective, the individual's concerns are converted into *clinical entities* that may be readily detached from the person who actually carries the weight of these problems. That is, by focusing on clinical problems, such as early satiety with weight loss, the pain and suffering of the individual living with the deformity may become displaced. It becomes easy to compartmentalize and put aside the real life perspective.

For instance, professionals focus on the high risk of fracture with falls, while individuals with osteoporosis may develop a profound fear of falling that inhibits life as it used to be. Likewise, professionals may focus on discomfort or pain related to vertebral collapse, while women describe feeling confined in a body contorted with pain—a body that has betrayed them, often abruptly and unexpectedly. The impact of physiological changes in the skeletal mass extend far beyond the bones.

LIVING WITH OSTEOPOROSIS: LOOKING BEYOND WHAT WE SEE

Stop for a moment and picture the image of a woman with osteoporosis. What descriptive words come to mind? Vibrant? Vital? Energetic? Capable? Probably not. More commonly, descriptors focus on frailty, deformity, weakness, or disability. Where have you seen this image before? Think back to the fairy tales and storybooks you read as a child . . . isn't this much like the picture of the wicked witch, or of the very, very old grandmother? Such negative portrayals often permeate the perceptions of women with osteoporosis. They feel as if they are assuming the shape of their elderly mothers, far before they reach old age. Others liken their image to the wicked witch, with jutting chin, a bony humped back, and seemingly long dangling arms. When accompanied by their husbands, these women may be mistaken for their mothers-in-law, or even their grandmothers! Think of this insult to self-esteem, added to the pain of living with osteoporosis.

In a poignant descriptive handbook written by Horner (1989), a woman with osteoporosis, the lived realities of these clinical entities pour forth. Having suffered several vertebral fractures, this woman endures the classic postural changes. She poignantly describes the way these changes make her feel.

When the spine shrinks so drastically, it causes the abdomen to protrude in a most unsightly fashion and the waistline completely disappears. This, coupled with a noticeable curvature of the upper spine, made me dread looking in the mirror. It was disconcerting, to say the least, to see the face and figure of my aged mother reflected there in place of the slim, straight me of a few short months ago. Even now, when exercise and increasing strength have enabled me to straighten up considerably, I shudder when I catch sight of my walking profile reflected in a store window. (p. 9)

She expounds on the clinical difficulty of eating, saying she would "force as much food as I could past the lump in my throat. Eating at any time was no great pleasure . . . " (p. 9). Imagine being told that any improvement would be so slow that there was no need to do densitometry more often than *annually* to assess the response, if any, to treatment. While that seems like a reasonable, cost-effective use of technology to professionals, hear the sting of those words on Horner's ears.

The doctors were understandably vague because it would be some months before they'd be able to determine whether the calcium drain had been arrested. And there would probably be no perceptible increase in bone mass for at least a year, if ever. In my darkest moments I'd visualize all my bones disintegrating until I dissolved into an amorphous mass and slithered out under the door! (p. 9)

The risk of falling was indelibly etched on her mind, " . . . when I first ventured outside on my own, I had an almost pathological fear of falling" (p. 9).

The high risk of fracture suddenly overshadows everyday life—dangerous situations abound. For example, functional reach increasingly becomes an issue. High cupboards or shelves that require a stretching, overhead reach (or, worse yet, a stepstool or ladder) pose significant concerns. Mobility and balance issues arise as uneven walking surfaces are encountered. We educate our clients in body mechanics to protect the spine and to prevent falls. We teach others to spot the danger zones and to intervene. But there is so much more to living with osteoporosis.

Many phenomena that we encounter in everyday life could become frightening, given the newly found threat of fall and fracture. We who do not have a fear of falling hop on and off escalators without much thought, maybe just a glance to check our footing when getting on and stepping off. But stop and think . . . the first step is critical—don't hit the crack or you may not be able to recover quickly enough, and a fall will follow. Then, the smooth surface of the entry step shifts as the step lifts, demanding a shift of weight distribution onto the emerging surface. Sharp, cutting edges of shiny metal protrude from the step edge like teeth, threatening to compound the injury of a fall. The railing provides some relief, but the width doesn't accommodate a small hand and its attachment won't permit a good grip. Where to focus the eyes . . . not on the moving metal, not on the moving images of the store displays, not on the distorted image in the mirrors lining the escalator, and certainly not into the eyes of the people watching and looking. . . . Finally the end is in sight; the step now begins to shrink away. New fear emerges—how will the off-step be? The gnawing metal teeth pull back and merge once again into a smooth metal surface. The exit ramp merges with sharp teeth of its own, now sucking the endless metal ramp into stillness. An awkward step, hoping to land squarely and to maintain balance as the inadequate (but welcomed) handrail slips off to continue its endless circle. Firm ground brings some relief once balance is restored—but don't stop here! There are people streaming from behind you, around both sides, impatiently stepping around the "slow old person."

Compound this event with a crowded shopping scene—people bumping, stepping in front, creating moving targets for rapid accommodation. For most women, there is also a handbag to manage, not to mention bags from purchases, too. Sometimes efforts to conceal or transfigure deformity actually make it worse. For example, a woman may select dress shoes with a modest heel over more sensible walking shoes. These potentially frightening scenes are encountered in so many common places—the people movers at airports or amusement parks; the darkened, sloping aisles in movie theaters; the uneven surface of walking trails; or even cracked and shifted sidewalks in older neighborhoods. Add to this mix the hazards of climate—snow, ice, or wet surfaces compound concerns. Living with osteoporosis presents new challenges—challenges that we seldom stop to consider, unless it becomes *our* turn.

ACCOMMODATIONS WITHIN THE FAMILY

The accommodations imposed on those who live with osteoporosis often intrude into family-role relations. What must it be like when grandma or grandpa can no longer lift the grandbabies? Or when a loving hug becomes dangerous to fragile bones? Consider how adult children may express newly founded concerns for safety. Perhaps, by being overly cautious, or maybe by scolding children or parents who undertake "risky" behaviors. Role relations may shift dramatically as a new sense of protective "watching over" invades the family.

Some well-meaning families act on their protectiveness by changing the home environment without seeking the affected person's consent. They seek to "fix" the environment, much like we clinicians do. How many times have you heard tales of throw rugs being lifted, then mysteriously reappearing? Or of people resorting to climbing on chairs when their favorite stepstool was removed?

Even loving acts can go astray when not implemented within a framework of open communication and consensus building. Accommodations reach *into life,* not merely into the stage within which life is played out. Therefore, changes must be negotiated and agreed on, rather than imposed externally. Before initiating accommodative changes, it is important to recall the multifaceted impact of osteoporosis. Such changes reach into a life in complex ways . . . consider these facets over and against the accommodations that are routinely prescribed and implemented to maximize functional capability and provide safety.

THE RESEARCH PERSPECTIVE

Tiffany (1988) conducted a phenomenological study of older women's experience of osteoporosis using Colaizzi's analytic method. Generally, the goal of this type of research is to describe the lived experience of a given phenomenon. Themes identified through careful reflective analysis of in-depth interviews are then woven into a composite narrative that exemplifies the experience.

In Tiffany's study, the experience of living with osteoporosis was represented in a number of themes aggregated around three domains: psychologic, social, and biologic. The psychologic domain incorporated isolation, depression, weight control, and isolation with creativity, a sense of humor, attitude and feelings. This domain exemplifies the opposing characteristics that emerge as these older women learned to live with osteoporosis, and somehow become integrated into a unified whole being of a woman with osteoporosis. The social domain gives clues as to the importance of establishing and drawing resources from a network of others. Living arrangements, family, help seeking, and information seeking emerged as prominent themes in this domain. Even in the biologic domain, themes such as heritage, pain, height loss, fall prevention, and mobility demonstrate how discrete physiological changes in bone permeate the lived experiences of these women in a much broader sense. The women in this study overcame transient feelings of being sick, ugly, or dependent, and emerged as women living life to its fullest.

Paier (1996) conducted a phenomenological study focused on the experiences of postmenopausal women who suffered vertebral fractures (also using Colaizzi's analytic technique). In this study, five major theme clusters were derived: grappling with the forces of pain, self-taught resilience, the specter of the crone, vulnerability and vigilance, and contingent hope. Abrupt, excruciating pain began with the fracture and, for many, continued long after. Pain intruded on life experience, described as a choreographer of activity, an isolator, and a helpful protector. Again, opposing characteristics become evident and are merged into a wholeness of being manifested by these women.

Resilience, described as self-taught, was developed through information seeking and trial and error. These women explored the incongruencies and got to know their changed bodies through experimentation with activity. The specter of the crone (i.e., a withered old woman) hovered over these women as they associated postural changes with older women they knew, and focused attentively on straightening their backs. A continued fear of fracture is revealed in perceived fragility and weighing risks of certain activities—the women became vulnerable and vigilant. Finally, a form of tentative hope contingent upon the efficacy of their lifestyle and treatment plan was balanced with opposing concerns about the uncertainty of the progression of the disease. Again, the women in this study actively pursued changes in how they lived their lives in order to minimize the threats posed by their porous bones. Clearly, the impact of osteoporosis goes much further than microscopic changes in the skeleton.

Other quantitative studies have focused on more theoretically discrete concepts. For example, Kim, Horan, Gendler, and Patel (1991) studied elderly women's perceptions of their risks of developing osteoporosis from the perspective of the health belief. Kessenich and Guyatt (1998) investigated health-related quality of life (HRQL) in women with osteoporotic vertebral fractures. They found that all of the five domains of HRQL measured (symptoms, physical function, activities of daily living, emotional function, and leisure) were impacted by osteoporotic changes. Echoing this sentiment, Gold et al. (1991) studied the effect of health locus of control (HLOC) on psychosocial adaptation. These findings, though limited, have important implications for improving the quality of life for individuals who have osteoporosis—likewise, however they remind us how much more we need to know in order to improve the lived experience for those who have osteoporosis.

CONCLUSIONS

Powerful anecdotal evidence tells us that osteoporosis has profound effects on how one lives his/her life. Qualitative research into the lived experiences of women with osteoporosis confirms these reports. *Micro*scopic skeletal changes affect life *macro*scopically. Yet, we don't understand the course of disablement experienced by people with osteoporosis. We know that fracture poses a significant transition, marked by pain and functional disablement. But we also know that despite this disablement, people with osteoporosis still manage to integrate opposing characteristics and feelings into a unique whole being that lives life to the fullest. What are the hallmarks of these success stories? How can we, as carers, facilitate such success? We know so much, yet have so much more to learn.

REFERENCES

Cooper, C., Campion, G., & Melton, L. J. III. (1992). Hip fractures in the elderly: A worldwide projection. *Osteoporosis International, 2,* 285–289.

Gold, D. T., Smith, S. D., Bales, C. W., Lyles, K. W., Westlund, R. E., & Drezner, M. K. (1991). Osteoporosis in late life: Does health locus of control affect psychosocial adaptation? *Journal of the American Geriatrics Society, 39,* 670–675.

Horner, P. (1989). *The long road back: One woman's story.* Ottawa, Canada: University of Ottawa Press.

Kessenich, C. R., & Guyatt, G. H. (1998). Domains of health-related quality of life in elderly women with osteoporosis. *Journal of Gerontological Nursing, 24,* 7–13.

Kim, K. K., Horan, M. L., Gendler, P., & Patel, M. K. L. (1991). Development and evaluation of the osteoporosis health belief scale. *Research in Nursing and Health, 14,* 155–163.

Magaziner, J., Simonsick, E. M., Kashner, M., Hebel, J. R., & Kenzora, J. E. (1990). Predictors of functional recovery one year following hospital discharge for hip fracture: A prospective study. *Journal of Gerontology, Medical Sciences, 45,* M101–M107.

Melton, L. J. III, Ilstrup, D. M., Riggs, B. L., & Beckenbaurg, R. D. (1982). Fifty-year trend in hip fracture incidence. *Clinical Orthopedics, 162,* 144–149.

Paier, G. S. (1996). Specter of the crone: The experience of vertebral fracture. *Advances in Nursing Science, 18*(3), 27–36.

Tiffany, J. E. (1988). *The older woman and the experience of osteoporosis.* Unpublished doctoral dissertation, Graduate School of the Texas Woman's University, College of Nursing, Denton, Texas.

4

Nutritional Considerations

Helen Smiciklas-Wright and Catherine E. Wright

Count on calcium.

—H. Smiciklas-Wright

Nutrition is an essential factor in the maintenance of bone health and the prevention and treatment of osteoporosis. Prevention and management of osteoporosis is critical at three stages:

- *Primary prevention*—acquiring bone mass
- *Secondary prevention*—conserving bone mass
- *Treatment*—arresting bone loss, replacing lost bone, facilitating recovery from fractures

Dietary factors can play a crucial role at all three stages. In this chapter, we will deal primarily with calcium, the most critical nutrient affecting bone mass, and with vitamin D, which is important in absorption and metabolism of calcium. We will also discuss the role of phytoestrogens, plant compounds that have weak estrogenic activity and so may decrease bone resorption. It should be kept in mind, however, that many other dietary factors also have an effect on bone health. Calcium is only one constituent of bone, and changes in bone mass cannot always be corrected by increasing the calcium supply. Nutritional factors that are known to be important for bone health are:

- Calcium
- Energy
- Phosphorus
- Vitamin D
- Protein
- Vitamin C
- Manganese
- Vitamin K
- Zinc
- Copper

The effect of other nutrients may be direct, as in the case of zinc, magnesium, and copper, which are essential cofactors for enzymes active in bone development. Other dietary factors may play a less direct role in maintaining bone health. Low energy intake, for example, can result in inadequate intakes of most other nutrients. Many older adults have reduced energy intakes, causing them to have low body muscle mass and weakness, and putting them at risk for falls and fractures.

CALCIUM

The role of calcium in reducing osteoporotic risk is not straightforward. There are inconsistencies among studies, challenges in assessing habitual calcium intake, and many other risk factors that may modulate the role of calcium in given individuals. Nevertheless, the findings from observational/ epidemiologic studies and randomized trials indicate that calcium plays an important role in achieving and maintaining bone mass.

Does Calcium Have an Effect on Peak Bone Mass?

Peak bone mass (i.e., the amount of bone predominantly acquired by young adulthood) is a significant determinant of future fracture risk. The peak bone mass that can be achieved is genetically determined; however, calcium intake affects whether this maximum is reached. A number of calcium supplementation studies have demonstrated gains in bone mineral density at various skeletal sites when diet and supplement provide about 1,500 mg of calcium daily (Andon, Lloyd, & Matkovic, 1994). However, the benefits of supplementation disappear after supplementation is withdrawn. It appears that calcium intakes need to be maintained throughout growth to result in a higher peak bone mass in adulthood (Institute of Medicine, 1997).

Can Calcium Decrease the Risk of Osteoporosis in Pre- and Postmenopausal Women?

In premenopausal women, adequate calcium intake and regular weight-bearing exercises go hand-in-hand in maintaining bone mass. The effectiveness of calcium supplements in postmenopausal women is of particular interest, given that a great deal of advertising is directed to these women. There is a growing body of evidence that increasing calcium intake can reduce bone loss (Reid, Ames, Evans, Gamble, & Sharpe, 1995) and the risk of fractures (Cumming & Nevitt, 1997).

An important question is whether calcium requirements are different for women who are undertaking hormone replacement therapy (HRT). Recently, Nieves, Komar, Cosman, and Lindsay (1998) reported that calcium potentiates the effect of estrogen and calcitonin on bone mass. The combined effect of calcium and estrogen was two- to three-fold greater than estrogen alone in reducing changes in bone mass. Thus, the calcium requirements of women on HRT may not be lower than those of other postmenopausal women. Calcium continues to be an important component in any regime to prevent and treat osteoporosis.

A critical issue is whether calcium intake can prevent fractures. One of the earliest studies was that of Matkovic et al. (1979), which found that the annual rate of hip fractures in rural Yugoslavian women was lower in one district, in which inhabitants habitually consumed dairy products, than in a second district, where average dairy intake was low. This and more recent studies (Cumming & Nevitt, 1997) support the recommendations that older women should increase their calcium intake.

Calcium Recommendations

The Institute of Medicine, National Academy of Science (NAS), recently published new requirements for calcium (Institute of Medicine, 1997) for the first time since 1989. The values of these Dietary Reference Intakes (DRI) for calcium are shown in Table 4.1. They are higher than the previous recommendations for most age groups. The recommendation for adults over age 50 is 1,200 mg, considerably higher than the 800 mg previously recommended. The new recommendations also endorse higher recommendations for adolescents. The new, higher recommendations are based on evidence supporting the importance of calcium to bone health across the lifespan.

How Much Calcium Do Americans Consume?

Most Americans do not consume the recommended amounts of calcium. Data from large nationwide surveys show that the average adult gets 500 to 800 mg of calcium per day from food sources; men, on the average, consume higher levels than women. Average intakes by gender and age, obtained during the 1994–1996 Nationwide Continuing Survey of Food Intake by Individuals (CSFII), are shown in Figure 4.1.

Meeting Calcium Requirements

Calcium is available in foods and supplements. Foods are generally better sources because they provide other nutrients important for overall health as well as bone health and may provide nutrients that enable calcium absorption and metabolism.

TABLE 4.1 Dietary Reference Intakes

Life stage	Calcium (mg/day)	Vitamin D (μg/day [IU])
Children		
4–8 yrs.	800	5 (200)
Males and females		
9–18 yrs.	1300	5 (200)
19–50 yrs.	1000	5 (200)
51–70 yrs.	1200	10 (400)
>70 yrs.	1200	15 (600)

Source: Institute of Medicine, 1997.

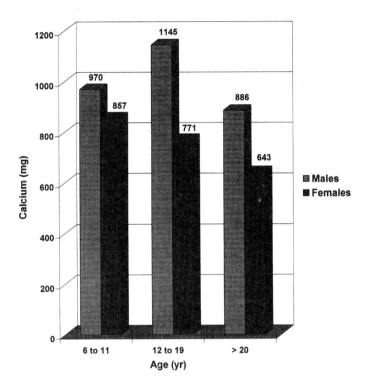

FIGURE 4.1   Mean intake of calcium by sex and age.

Source: USDA Continuing Survey of Food Intakes by Individuals, 1994–1996.

Dairy Products

Traditionally, dairy products have been the most calcium-rich foods. Dairy products are readily available, convenient, and reasonably priced. Calcium in milk is readily absorbed because milk is fortified with vitamin D, which facilitates calcium absorption. The approximate calcium content of commonly used dairy products is shown in Table 4.2. Lower-fat milks contain more calcium than regular milk because some nonfat milk products are added to replace the fat. Cottage cheese has traditionally been considered a relatively poor dairy source of calcium because calcium is lost during production. However, some cottage cheese and even some milk are fortified with calcium.

TABLE 4.2 Approximate Amount of Calcium in Dairy Products

Food	Amount	Calcium (mg)
Nonfat milk	1 c.	415
Whole milk	1 c.	315
Milk, Ca fortified	1 c.	500
Yogurt	1 c.	300
Dry skim milk powder	1/4 c.	210
Cheddar, other hard cheeses	1 oz.	150
Parmesan, grated	2 T.	150
Ice cream	1/2 c.	85
Cottage cheese	1/2 c.	70
Cottage cheese, Ca fortified	1/2 c.	200

Barriers to Dairy Product Use

Per capita consumption of milk has declined in the past 25 years. Many people prefer the taste of other beverages to that of milk or choose noncaloric beverages for the purposes of weight control. Girls, especially, tend to worry that milk will make them "fat" (Novotny, Han, & Biernacke, 1999).

Lactose intolerance is a major reason for avoiding dairy products. Lactose intolerance occurs in people who have insufficient levels of the intestinal enzyme lactase to break down lactose, the principle carbohydrate in milk. Lactose that is not well digested can undergo microbial fermentation. The consequent gastrointestinal symptoms (i.e., bloating, cramps, pain, and diarrhea) may be mild or severe. Some people with real or perceived lactose intolerance choose to restrict and even eliminate dairy products from their diets.

New research indicates that many people who have symptoms of lactose intolerance can tolerate small amounts of dairy products without experiencing gastrointestinal discomfort (McBean & Miller, 1998). Solid products, such as cheese, may be better tolerated because of delayed gastric emptying time. Yogurts with active cultures and hard cheeses have lower lactose contents. Drinking milk with other foods and the addition of chocolate to milk are two ways to improve lactose intolerance. Lactose-reduced milks are also available but are more expensive than regular milk.

Nondairy Food Sources

There are two categories of nondairy food sources that provide calcium: those that naturally contain calcium and those that are fortified with calcium.

The values in Table 4.3 show that calcium is present in varying amounts in a wide range of foods. There are some good sources of calcium in vegetables, such as kale, collard greens, and Chinese cabbage, with lesser amounts in broccoli, green beans, and acorn squash. Spinach is a good source but contains oxalic acid, which binds the calcium in spinach and interferes with its absorption. Phytic acid in dried peas and beans can also decrease calcium absorption. Canned sardines, salmon, and mackerel are excellent sources of calcium. As more and more foods are fortified, the number of good calcium sources increases. Some manufacturers produce calcium fortified rice, prune juice, pasta, waffles, and other foods. Reading food labels becomes evermore important for determining calcium intake.

Interpreting Food Labels

As more calcium-fortified foods appear in food markets, it is helpful to read food labels to know how much calcium is in a food product. However, interpreting a food label requires some information that is not on the label. The calcium content of foods is listed as a percent Daily Value (DV). For example, the amount of calcium in a fortified hot cereal is shown as 15% DV. To interpret this and estimate the amount of calcium (mg) in the cereal, one needs to know that the DV for calcium is currently set at 1,000 mg.

TABLE 4.3 Approximate Amount of Calcium in Nondairy Food Products

Food	Amount	Calcium (mg)
Sardines, canned, drained	4 oz.	425
Salmon, canned, drained	1/2 c.	240
Mackerel, canned drained	1/2 c.	240
Cereal, super-fortified	1/2 c.	170
Oatmeal, instant	1 pkg.	165
Orange juice, Ca fortified	1/2 c.	140
Chinese cabbage, cooked	1/2 c.	80
Kale, cooked	1/2 c.	90
Tofu, firm processed with Ca	1/4 c.	65
Broccoli	1/2 c.	50
Orange	1	50
Beans, lima, kidney, navy	1/2 c.	40
Egg, large	1	2
Bread, white	1 slice	25

Thus, the cereal with 15% DV calcium per serving would contain 150 mg of calcium.

CALCIUM SUPPLEMENTS

Supplements are available as a number of salt forms, which can differ in their elemental calcium content as well as their solubility (see Table 4.4).

The most common and generally least expensive form of calcium is calcium carbonate. This includes well-known products such as Tums and the recently available Viactive, which is a chewable "candy." Calcium carbonate contains the highest amount of calcium of any salt so the dosages are smaller. If it is convenient, calcium carbonate supplements are best taken with meals to increase calcium absorption. Calcium citrate supplements have less calcium but are acidic and may be better for older people with reduced stomach acidity. All supplements can be taken in several small doses across the day for the most efficient calcium absorption.

Some people complain that calcium supplements cause constipation, bloating, or gastric irritation. Physicians usually recommend trying another type of supplement to relieve the symptoms.

Does Excess Caffeine Affect Bone?

High caffeine consumption has been suggested as a risk factor for osteoporosis. Various physiological mechanisms have been proposed to account for the risk. Unfortunately, studies of caffeine consumption (coffee supplies most of the caffeine in Western diets) as a potential risk factor have been

TABLE 4.4 Calcium Content of Supplements

Supplement/salt	Milligrams of calcium in 1 gram tablet
Calcium carbonate	400
Dicalcium phosphate	230
Calcium citrate	180
Calcium lactate	130
Bonemeal	300
Dolomite	200

contradictory. Overall, the evidence suggests that daily caffeine intake equivalent to about two or three servings of brewed coffee may increase bone loss in women with low calcium intake. However, the bone loss was shown to be insignificant in women with adequate calcium intake (Harris & Dawson-Hughes, 1994).

Does Excess Protein Affect Bone?

The concern about high protein intake comes from many studies done over many years that show that urinary calcium excretion increases as protein intake increases (Heaney, 1993). The issue of protein intake is clearly important since protein is necessary for bone as well as muscle, and low protein intake depresses calcium absorption. Massey (1998) has emphasized the importance of protein for elderly persons who are at most risk for fractures.

There is no simple answer to the question, "Does high protein intake adversely affect bone?" It really does depend on the amount of calcium consumed and what else in the diet can buffer some of the renal consequences of a high acid-ash diet. Meat, fish, and cheese produce high potential renal acid loads (Barzel & Massey, 1998), and older adults may be more sensitive to acidic diets. However, vegetables, fruits, milk, and yogurts supply an alkali-ash diet, which buffers diets rich in acid-ash. This is one of many arguments for a varied diet with adequate servings from each of the food groups.

VITAMIN D

Calcium deficiency is not the only cause of brittle bones. In many older adults, a deficiency of vitamin D may also be to blame. The role of vitamin D is to maintain the serum levels of calcium and phosphorus within a specific range. Vitamin D enhances the efficiency of absorption of dietary calcium and phosphorus and mobilizes stores of these minerals from bone if their serum concentrations drop below a certain level.

Vitamin D is not, in the true sense of the word, a vitamin; that is, it does not need to be supplied by dietary sources. It exists in the epidermis as a provitamin, which is converted to vitamin D upon exposure to light (Norman, 1998). In northern latitudes, during the summer months, 10 to

15 minutes of sun exposure two or three times per week should be sufficient to ensure adequate production of vitamin D in children and young adults. In winter months, it is often not possible to get enough vitamin D from sun exposure.

For several reasons, older adults are at risk of insufficient production of vitamin D. In the first place, the concentration of the provitamin in the epidermis decreases with age: older adults produce three to four times less vitamin D than young adults exposed to the same amount of sunlight. Furthermore, older adults often spend less time outdoors and thus have less exposure to sunlight than children and young adults. Nursing home residents, in particular, spend little time in the sun. One study of institutionalized and free-living elderly women found lower levels of vitamin D metabolites and calcium absorption in the former group (Kinyamu, Gallagher, Balhorn, & Petranick, 1997). Additionally, fear of skin cancer may cause older adults to be particularly conscientious about applying sunscreen, which hinders vitamin D production (sunscreen with a sun protection factor [SPF] of 8 or above almost completely blocks the production of vitamin D).

Vitamin D can also be obtained from dietary sources. However, many adults drink little milk, which is the only food that is routinely fortified with vitamin D. Aging itself does not alter vitamin D absorption, but older adults may also be more likely to suffer from diseases that cause intestinal malabsorption disorders (e.g., liver disease and Crohn's disease) and so be less able to absorb vitamin D.

Vitamin D deficiency in adults is known to lead to a skeletal mineralization defect causing osteomalacia. However, the role of vitamin D in preventing loss of bone mass and preserving bone strength is still under review. Some researchers have found that bone loss is reduced in older women given vitamin D supplements (Dawson-Hughes, Dallal, Krall, Harris, Sokol, & Falconer, 1991); other studies have found no connection between vitamin D intake and bone mass or hip fracture incidence (Lips, Graafmans, Ooms, Bezemer, & Bouter, 1996; Sowers, Wallace, Hollis, & Lemke, 1986). Associations may not be apparent in persons with reasonably adequate vitamin D status prior to supplementation.

Recommendations and Sources

Recommendations for vitamin D are hard to establish because the amount required depends on the level of vitamin D synthesized through exposure to sunlight. However, synthesis of vitamin D is affected by season of the year, time of day, latitude, skin pigmentation, and amount of clothing and sunscreen worn (Institute of Medicine, 1997). The current recommendations for vitamin D intake are shown in Table 4.1. The recommendations are shown both in micrograms (ug) and International Units (IU) and are highest for older adults.

Diet is the most reliable source of vitamin D in temperate zones. While many animal foods such as milk, eggs, butter, fish, and liver oils contain some vitamin D, it is generally difficult to get the recommended amounts from unfortified foods.

In the United States and Canada, milk is the only food that is routinely fortified with vitamin D. Most milk sold in North America is fortified to provide 100 IU per 8 oz. This is shown in the milk label as 25% DV per serving; the DV for vitamin D is 400 IU. However, several recent surveys revealed that not all milk samples analyzed had the expected amount of vitamin D. Other products such as cereals may also be vitamin D fortified.

IS IT POSSIBLE TO CONSUME TOO MUCH CALCIUM AND VITAMIN D?

Both calcium and vitamin D can cause health risks when consumed in very high amounts. The Institute of Medicine, the National Academy of Science (Institute of Medicine, 1997), recently set upper limits (ULs) for both calcium and vitamin D for persons one year old and older: UL for calcium = 2,500 mg/day, UL for vitamin D = 50 ug (2,000 IU)/day.

The potential risks of high calcium intake are decreased absorption of other minerals such as iron and zinc that can compete for absorption sites with calcium and formation of kidney stones. The risk of kidney stones is a complex issue because there are many causes of renal stones.

The potential risk of excessive vitamin D intake is damage to target tissues such as those of the central nervous system, which can result in severe depression, nausea, and anorexia.

It is unlikely that people would consume toxic levels of calcium and vitamin D from traditional food sources. However, with the increasing availability of supplements and fortified foods, it will be important to monitor intakes of these nutrients.

PHYTOESTROGENS

Incidence of osteoporosis shows wide geographical variation. Despite the linkage between calcium intake and bone health, osteoporosis incidence is low in many areas, particularly in developing countries, where calcium intake is also low. There are many possible explanations for this apparent paradox:

- Differential reporting—osteoporosis rates may simply be underrepresented in some areas.
- Life expectancies—the longer life expectancies of people in developed countries may lead to a greater risk of osteoporosis.
- Nondietary factors—genetic differences, exercise patterns, exposure to sunlight/vitamin D production, etc.
- Other dietary factors

Among dietary components that may affect bone strength, soy products are of interest. In Asian countries, where rates of osteoporosis have been low, large amounts of soy products are consumed (Barrett, 1996).

There are three possible ways in which consumption of soy may contribute to bone health (Messina, 1995). In the first place, soy protein causes less calcium to be excreted in urine than animal protein; thus, consumption of soy products in place of meat may lead to retention of calcium. Second, some soy products themselves contain calcium. Third, soy contains several compounds that are classified as phytoestrogens (Dwyer et al., 1994). Phytoestrogens are plant compounds that structurally resemble estrogens; when eaten, they may have estrogenic effects. Evidence from animal studies shows that phytoestrogens are effective in stimulating bone mineralization and preventing bone loss (Adlercreutz & Mazur, 1997). While phytoestrogens have not been proven to prevent osteoporosis in humans, phytoestrogen-containing foods (soy products, whole grain cereals, seeds, berries, and nuts) may be effective in maintaining bone health.

SUMMARY

There is a persuasive body of evidence that nutritional factors play significant roles in development and maintenance of bone strength. Calcium has been the most extensively studied nutritional factor and appears to be important in bone integrity throughout life. Other dietary factors, vitamin D, energy, protein, micronutrients, and phytoestrogens can all have significant roles to play in reducing osteoporotic risk.

REFERENCES

Adlercreutz, H., & Mazur, W. (1997). Phyto-oestrogens and western diseases. *Annals of Medicine, 29,* 95–120.

Andon, M. B., Lloyd, T., & Matkovic, V. (1994). Supplementation trials with calcium citrate malate: Evidence in favor of increasing the calcium RDA during childhood and adolescence. *Journal of Nutrition, 124,* 412S–417S.

Barrett, J. (1996). Phytoestrogens: Friends or foes? *Environmental Health Perspectives, 104,* 478–482.

Barzel, U. S., & Massey, L. K. (1998). Excess dietary protein can adversely affect bone. *Journal of Nutrition, 128,* 1051–1053.

Cumming, R. G., & Nevitt, M. C. (1997). Calcium for prevention of osteoporotic fractures in post-menopausal women. *Journal of Bone and Mineral Research, 12,* 1321–1329.

Dawson-Hughes, B., Dallal, G. E., Krall, E. A., Harris, S., Sokol, L. J., & Falconer, G. (1991). Effect of vitamin D supplementation on wintertime and overall bone loss on healthy postmenopausal women. *Annals of Internal Medicine, 125,* 505–512.

Dwyer, J. T., Goldin, B. R., Saul, N., Gualtirei, L., Barakat, S., & Adlerkruetz, H. (1994). Tofu and soy drinks contain phytoestrogens. *Journal of the American Dietetic Association, 94,* 739–743.

Harris, S. S., & Dawson-Hughes, B. (1994). Caffeine and bone loss in healthy postmenopausal women. *American Journal of Clinical Nutrition, 60,* 573–578.

Heaney, R. P. (1993). Protein intake and the calcium economy. *Journal of the American Dietetic Association, 93,* 125–160.

Institute of Medicine (IOM). (1997). *Dietary reference intakes for calcium, phosphorus, magnesium, vitamin D, and fluoride.* Standing Committee on the Scientific Evaluation of Dietary Reference Intakes. Food and Nutrition Board. Washington, DC: National Academy Press.

Kinyamu, H. K., Gallagher, J. C., Balhorn, K. E., & Petranick, K. M. (1997). Serum vitamin D metabolism and calcium absorption in normal young and elderly free-living women and in women living in nursing homes. *American Journal of Clinical Nutrition, 65,* 790–797.

Lips, P., Graafmans, W. C., Ooms, M. E., Bezemer, P. D., & Bouter, L. M. (1996). Vitamin D supplementation and fracture incidence in elderly persons. *American College of Physicians, 124,* 400–406.

Massey, L. K. (1998). Does excess dietary protein adversely affect bone? *Journal of Nutrition, 128,* 1048–1050.

Matkovic, V., Kostial, K., Siminovic, I., Buzina, R., Brodarec, A., & Nordin, B. E. (1979). Bone status and fracture rates in two regions of Yugoslavia. *American Journal of Clinical Nutrition, 32,* 540–549.

McBean, L. D., & Miller, G. D. (1998). Allaying fears and fallacies about lactose intolerance. *Journal of the American Dietetic Association, 98,* 671–676.

Messina, M. (1995). Modern applications for an ancient bean: Soybeans and the prevention and treatment of chronic disease. *Journal of Nutrition, 125,* 567S–569S.

Nieves, J. W., Komar, L., Cosman, F., & Lindsay, R. (1998). Calcium potentiates the effect of estrogen and calcitonin on bone mass: Review and analysis. *American Journal of Clinical Nutrition, 67,* 18–24.

Norman, A. W. (1998). Sunlight, season, skin, pigmentation, vitamin D, and 25-hydroxyvitamin D: Integral components of the vitamin D endocrine system. *American Journal of Clinical Nutrition, 67,* 1108–1110.

Novotny, R., Han, J.-S., & Biernacke, I. (1999). Motivators and barriers to consuming calcium-rich foods among Asian adolescents in Hawaii. *Journal of Nutrition Education, 31,* 99–104.

Reid, I. R., Ames, R. W., Evans, M. C., Gamble, G. D., & Sharpe S. J. (1995). Long-term effects of calcium supplementation, bone loss and fractures in postmenopausal women: A randomized controlled trial. *American Journal of Medicine, 98,* 331–335.

Sowers, M. R., Wallace, R. B., Hollis, B. W., & Lemke, J. H. (1986). Parameters related to 25-OH-D levels in a population-based study of women. *American Journal of Clinical Nutrition, 43,* 621–628.

5

Exercise: A Prescription for Osteoporosis?

Susan Rankin

Exercise—Giving up a half-hour (one sitcom) of TV is all
it takes.

—S. Rankin

Previous chapters in this book indicate that individuals with osteoporosis are at an increased risk of fracture due to a net loss of bone mass.
The cellular mechanisms causing decreased bone mass are increased
osteoclast-mediated bone resorption and/or decreased osteoblast-mediated
bone formation. The authors indicated in their discussions that bone loss
can be prevented by hormone replacement therapy and nutritional supplementation. Weight-bearing activities and muscle strength/endurance exercise programs also play a role in retarding bone loss and are the focus of
this chapter. After reading this chapter the reader will (a) understand the
effects of exercise regimes on skeletal health and (b) identify exercise
prescriptions for various populations (e.g., osteoporotic vs. nonosteoporotic)
to improve skeletal health.

The initial section of the chapter will discuss the effects of immobilization
on bone and review bone architecture. Next, a review of the literature

regarding peak bone mass and the effect of exercise programs on bone mass will be reviewed. Finally, suggested exercise prescriptions will be presented for both the prevention of osteoporosis and for those already suffering from the disease.

EFFECTS OF DISUSE ON BONE MASS

Long periods of immobilization, weightlessness, paralysis, and recumbancy result in demineralization of the skeleton. This is due to unrestrained osteoclast-mediated bone resorption and decreased osteoblast-mediated bone formation. In a review of the studies focusing on disuse, immobilized limbs of dogs (Uhthoff & Jaworski, 1978), turkeys (Rubin & Lanyon, 1985), and monkeys (Young, Niklowits, Brown, & Jee, 1986) suggested loss of bone at the periosteal, endocortical, and trabecular surfaces, leading to thinning of both cortical and trabecular bone. The cortical bone also becomes more porous.

In the research conducted on human samples, comparable results were reported. For example, Westlin (1974) noted that women who had experienced a Colles' fracture sustained significant decreases in radial and ulnar bone density following four months in a forearm cast.

Research examining the effects of weightlessness on bone density yielded similar results. Crewman from Gemini flights IV, V, and VII experienced calcaneous, radial, and ulnar losses ranging from 2%–15%, 3%–25%, and 3%–16%, respectively (Mack, LaChance, Vose, & Vogt, 1967). During space flight when gravitational stress is absent, alterations of muscle structure become evident within the first week (Rock & Fortney, 1984). Since the integrity of bone is dependent upon the forces exerted upon it by the attached muscles, it is suggested that the decrease in muscular force applied to bone, along with the absence of gravity, accounts for the loss of bone during space flight.

Paralysis and extended recumbancy also result in a reduction in bone mass. Following paralysis, bone is initially lost from the entire skeleton. Later, bone loss selectively occurs from the paralyzed area (Claus-Walker & Halstead, 1982). Continuous bed rest also results in bone loss. For example, Schneider and McDonald (1984) observed calcaneal mineral losses averaging 5% per month in 90 healthy young men recumbent for 5 to 36 weeks. LeBlanc et al. (1987) noted that six healthy men at bed rest for five weeks lost a mean of 0.9% spinal bone mineral per week. Krolner and Toft's

(1983) results indicated a 0.9% loss of spinal bone per week in 17 women and 17 men confined to bed rest for disc protrusion.

The pattern for bone loss in disuse is similar to that in osteoporosis due to postmenopausal status, calcium deficiency (Recker, 1992), and excess glucorticoid states (Marcus, 1992). Previous chapters have indicated the amount of bone loss due to postmenopausal status. To review, the initial magnitude of bone loss is 3%–4% in one month (Chestnut, 1993) with total losses as high as 30%–50% (Uhthoff & Jaworski, 1978). What is the effect of weight-bearing exercise on bone integrity?

BONE ARCHITECTURE

Functional strain experienced by bone can be measured by using implanted strain gauges. Because peak functional strains in vertebrates are similar regardless of the size of the animal (Allen, 1994), and studies in humans pose some risk, animal models have been used to better understand the effects of exercise on bone structure (Recker, 1992; Rubin & Lanyon, 1985). When animals are exposed to loading stress, bone formation increases in the periosteum, endocortical, and trabecular surfaces. Although it is not possible to conclude from these studies the exercise requirements for humans, it is suggested that minimal loading can minimize bone loss (Allen, Pead, Skerry, & Lanyon, 1988; Rubin & Lanyon, 1984; Turner, Forwood, Rho, & Yoshikawa, 1994). The next section of this chapter will discuss peak bone mass and the effects of exercise programs on attaining and or maintaining bone mass.

PEAK BONE MASS

The two main determinants of bone mineral density are the magnitudes of peak bone mass achieved and bone lost. Peak bone mass is a major determinant of bone mass later in life (Hui, Slemenda, & Johnston, 1990), and an increase in peak bone mass may decrease the risk of osteoporotic fractures. Genetic factors play a major part in the determination of peak bone mass (Slemenda, Christian, Williams, Norton, & Johnston, 1991), accounting for nearly 80% of the variance. Still, 20% or more may be due to environmental factors, including nutrition and exercise. Since the research suggests that prevention is the cornerstone for managing osteoporosis, consideration of nutritional and lifestyle factors affecting the acquisition of peak bone mass and those affecting bone loss in the premenopausal and postmenopausal years needs to be examined.

Premenopausal bone mass is related to both physical activity (Aloia, Vaswani, Yeh, & Cohn, 1988; Slemenda, Miller, Hui, Reister, & Johnston, 1991) and calcium intake (Johnston et al., 1992). Exercise plays a role in the development of peak bone mass. Present studies indicate that peak mass is attained by the end of (Gilsanz et al., 1988) or soon after (Stevenson, Lees, Davenport, Cust, & Ganger, 1989) linear skeletal growth is complete. For example, Slemenda, Miller, et al. (1991) examined the association between the number of hours spent in weight bearing or nonweight-bearing activities and bone density at various sites in 118 children between the ages of 5.3 and 14 years. The results suggest that more active children may have a bone density that is 5%–10% greater than less active children. While it is suggested that physical activity may contribute to greater peak bone mass, it is also important to note that female athletes who participate in extreme exercise may become amenorrheic and are at risk for osteoporosis (Drinkwater et al., 1984; Hetland, Haarbo, & Christensen, 1993; Wolman, Clark, McNally, Harries, & Reeve, 1990).

As noted, peak bone mass is also a result of nutritional considerations. The research suggests that persons who consume greater quantities of calcium early in life have greater bone mass in later life (Halioua & Anderson, 1989; Matkovic et al., 1979; Sandler et al., 1985). In a more recent three-year, double-blind, placebo-controlled trial in prepubertal twins, Johnston et al. (1992) indicated that additional calcium (more than the current RDA of 1,200 mg) increased the rate of gain in skeletal mineral in children. Johnston concluded that if the gain persists, peak bone mass should be increased and the risk of postmenopausal fracture reduced.

Effects of Exercise Programs on Bone Mass

More than 30 cross-sectional and 20 prospective exercise studies focusing on the effect of exercise on bone mass have been published in the last decade (Drinkwater, 1993; Geusens & Dequeker, 1993; Gutin & Kasper, 1992; Martin & Novelovitz, 1993; Prince et al., 1991). These investigations varied with respect to sample size, menopausal status, age, body size, type of exercise including load intensity and duration, physical activity, aerobic fitness, bone site(s) measured, and method used to measure bone density.

The studies indicate that exercise programs in general improve bone mass or prevent bone loss (Allen, 1994).

It is clear from the research that weight-bearing activity is an important component of the exercise strategy. Resistive mechanical loading of the appendicular skeleton (Ayalon, Simkin, Leichter, & Raifmann, 1987) results in a positive effect on each respective site. Investigations using either "physical activity," e.g., daily energy expenditure estimates (Aloia, Cohn, Ostuni, Cane, & Ellis, 1978; Nelson, Fisher, Dilmanian, Dallal, & Evans, 1991; Oyster, Morton, & Linnell, 1984; Sinaki & Offord, 1988; Zhang, Feldbaum, & Fortney, 1992) or aerobic fitness expressed as maximal oxygen uptake or aerobic capacity (Pocock et al., 1989; Martin & Novelovitz, 1993), both correlate positively with bone mass.

As previously discussed, bone remodeling is influenced by mechanical stress. Trabeculae will develop in the direction of applied stress and will increase or decrease in size and number depending on the amount of stress. Muscle contractions stress the bones to which they are attached and muscle strength is related directly to its cross-sectional area (Frontera & Meredith, 1989; Rogers & Evans, 1993). This relationship is important because muscle strength has been associated with improved bone mass in top-ranked athletes (Nilsson & Westlin, 1971), premenopausal women (Pocock et al., 1989), and postmenopausal women (Sinaki, 1989; Sinaki & Offord, 1988; Halle, Schmidt, O'Dwyer, & Lin, 1990; Zimmerman, Schmidt, Brooks, Kinsey, & Eekhoff, 1990). The studies suggest that muscle mass and muscle strength are important to skeletal health. Bone loss with aging may be mediated by greater skeletal loading through increased muscle mass and strength (Aniansson & Gustavson, 1981; Brown, McCartnet, & Sale, 1990; Charette et al., 1991; Frontera, Meredith, O'Reilly, & Evans, 1988; Menkes et al., 1993; Nelson et al., 1991). Since the research evidence suggests that bone strength and muscle mass have a positive association, a short review of the literature on resistance training programs with older adults is provided.

RESISTANCE TRAINING PROGRAMS FOR OLDER ADULTS

Pyka, Lindberger, Charette, and Marcus (1994) studied the effects of resistance training on muscle strength and size in older people (17 women and 8 men, mean age 68 in 1-year study, randomly assigned). The results suggest that prolonged moderate- to high-intensity training may be carried out by healthy older adults with reasonable compliance and that such training leads to sustained increases in muscle strength. These improvements are rapidly achieved and are accompanied by hypertrophy of both Type 1 and Type 2 fibers. In a human cadaver study, Doyle, Brown, and LaChance (1970) noted that a significant correlation $(r = .72)$ existed between a measure of BMC of the third lumbar vertebral body and the weight of the left psoas muscle. Further, Pogrund, Bloom, and Weinberg (1986) reported a significant relationship $(r = .67)$ existed between psoas width and bone mass in the third lumbar vertebra in men and women ages 55 to 84 years. Subjects with narrow psoas widths demonstrated low lumbar bone mass levels.

SUMMARY

It is evident based on the research results that exercise is a viable strategy for the management of osteoporosis. However, the impact of exercise is greater when used in concert with other treatment modalities. For example, postmenopausal women who exercise and who are treated with estrogen have greater increases in bone mineral density than women in an estrogen-deficient state (Martin & Novelovitz, 1993; Prince et al., 1991). The research also suggests that to optimize the effect of an exercise program, calcium supplementation is encouraged (Prince et al., 1991). One additional benefit is that research results also indicate that exercise may improve calcium absorption which, as noted in previous chapters, will assist in the maintenance of bone integrity (Nelson, Meredith, Dawson-Hughes, & Evans, 1988; Nelson et al., 1991).

Another factor influencing the effects of exercise on bone integrity is that exercise effects are generally regional. For example, weight-bearing exercise can increase the density of the lower extremities and axial skeleton but not the upper extremities (Dalsky et al., 1988; Nelson et al., 1991). It is also important to note that the increased bone density realized from an exercise program are rapidly lost with detraining (Dalsky et al., 1988). The next section will provide suggested exercise prescriptions for the prevention of osteoporosis in healthy individuals and for those persons already suffering from the disease.

EXERCISE PRESCRIPTION FOR OSTEOPOROSIS

Before initiating any exercise program, the following prerequisites are essential. First, a physical assessment is highly recommended for anyone over

45 years of age. This assessment should consist of the following in regards to bone health. Musculoskeletal and cardiovascular status should be assessed. Muscle strength, endurance tests, and cardiovascular fitness tests should be administered. For example, grip strength correlates with back strength and may be used as a simple, inexpensive, and safe means of assessing back strength (Kritz-Silverstein & Barrett, 1994; Sinaki, 1989). A submaximal stress test based on ACSM guidelines (Blair et al., 1991) can be used to assess cardiovascular fitness.

The next part of the assessment will identify the risk factors associated with osteoporosis. If one or more of the risk factors predisposing an individual to osteoporosis are present, a bone density screening is suggested (see Table 5.1). Finally, based on the research regarding exercise programming and

TABLE 5.1 Who's at Risk?

Risk	Description
Age	Age increases the risk of developing osteoporosis. Bones become less dense and weaker with age.
Gender	Women are at a higher risk of developing osteoporosis than men. Women have less bone tissue and lose bone more rapidly due to the changes involved in menopause.
Race	Caucasian and Asian women are more likely to develop osteoporosis. However, African American and Hispanic women are also at significant risk for developing the disease.
Bone structure and body weight	Small-boned and thin women are at greater risk.
Menopause/ menstrual history	Normal or early menopause (brought about naturally or because of surgery) increases the risk of developing osteoporosis. In addition, women who stop menstruating before menopause, because of conditions such as anorexia or bulimia or because of excessive physical exercise, may also lose bone tissue and develop osteoporosis.
Lifestyle	Smoking, drinking too much alcohol, consuming an inadequate amount of calcium, or getting little or no weight-bearing exercise increases the risk of developing osteoporosis.
Medications and disease	Osteoporosis is associated with certain medications (e.g., cortisone-like drugs) and is a recognized complication of a number of medical conditions, including endocrine disorders (having an overactive thyroid), rheumatoid arthritis, and immobilization.
Family history	Genetic factors may increase the risk of developing osteoporosis.

Source: Adapted from the National Osteoporosis Foundation (http://www.nof.org).

other treatment modalities, adequate calcium supplementation and hormone replacement therapy are suggested if there are no contraindications.

Once the assessment is successfully completed, one may begin the osteoporosis exercise program. The program will vary based on the bone health of the individual. In the following two sections, the exercise prescription for osteoporosis prevention and for osteoporotic individuals will be presented.

Exercise Program for Osteoporosis Prevention

The program will follow the outline provided in Table 5.2. One should choose a weight-bearing activity that is enjoyable (walking, dancing, golf, racquet sports) and perform the site-specific exercise provided in Figures 5.1 and 5.2. These sites were chosen because of the increased risk of fracture at these sites. The exercises are to be performed following the *FIT* principle that is depicted in Table 5.3.

Exercise Program for Established Osteoporosis

In osteoporotic patients, the bone is very porous with a great decrease in trabecular structure. Therefore, in established osteoporosis, exercise is

TABLE 5.2 Osteoporosis Prevention Program

Type of activity	Description
Warm-up	5 minutes of brisk walking
	Flexibility program (series of stretches)
Site-specific strengthening exercises	Hip
	Pelvis
	Humerus
	Wrist
	Vertebra
	Rib
Weight-bearing activity	Walking
	Dancing
	Golf
	Racquet sports (squash, tennis, racquetball)
	Cross country skiing
Cool-down	Slower intensity of activity
	Repeat flexibility program

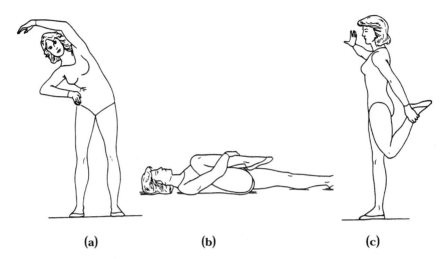

(a)   **(b)**   **(c)**

FIGURE 5.1 The preventative home program: Stretching examples.

Note: From *Osteoporosis: A guide to prevention and treatment* (pp. 147–155), by J. Aloia, 1989, Champaign, IL: Leisure Press. Copyright 1989 by Leisure Press. Reprinted with permission.

TABLE 5.3 FIT Program for Osteoporosis Prevention Program

FIT	Description
Frequency	3–5 times per week
Intensity (as determined by submaximal cardiovascular assessment)	Start at 40% of maximum aerobic capacity Progress to 70% of maximum aerobic ca- pacity
Time	Start with 15–20 minutes and gradually in- crease to 40 minutes

recommended but should be undertaken with extreme caution. In performing an exercise program, osteoporotic individuals should heed the following recommendations:

- Avoid flexion exercises (bending forward or sit-ups). Back flexion exercises may place an osteoporotic client at risk for vertebral compression fractures (Sinaki & Mikkelsen, 1984)
- Recommend isometric exercises for abdominal strengthening (Bartelink, 1957) and back extension (Sinaki, 1982)

- Restrict lifting to under 10 pounds
- Restrict any activities with components of twisting causing torque, such as golf and tennis
- Encourage postural training to maintain the spine in extension

Swimming is recommended as a means to increase cardiovascular endurance. Though swimming is not considered a weight-bearing exercise, deconditioned individuals will benefit initially from a swimming program by improving aerobic capacity and muscle strength. Figures 5.3 and 5.4 provide examples of site-specific exercises for individuals with established osteoporosis.

CONCLUSIONS

Currently, osteoporosis is a condition that is more amenable to prevention than treatment. Based on the research reviewed in this chapter, an exercise component should be included in a premenopausal prevention plan. In addition to calcium supplementation and hormone therapy, the literature also suggests that exercise should be one of the treatment modalities for patients with postmenopausal osteoporosis. In both cases, site-specific resistance training and weight-bearing activities appear to be beneficial.

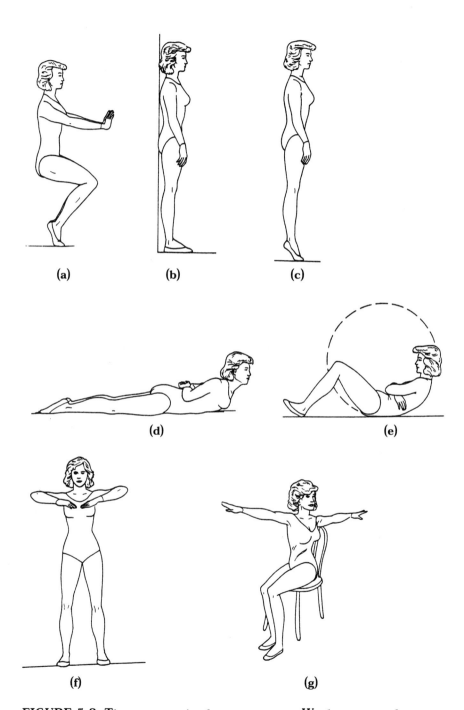

FIGURE 5.2 The preventative home program: Workout examples.

Note: From *Osteoporosis: A guide to prevention and treatment* (pp. 147–155), by J. Aloia, 1989, Champaign, IL: Leisure Press. Copyright 1989 by Leisure Press. Reprinted with permission.

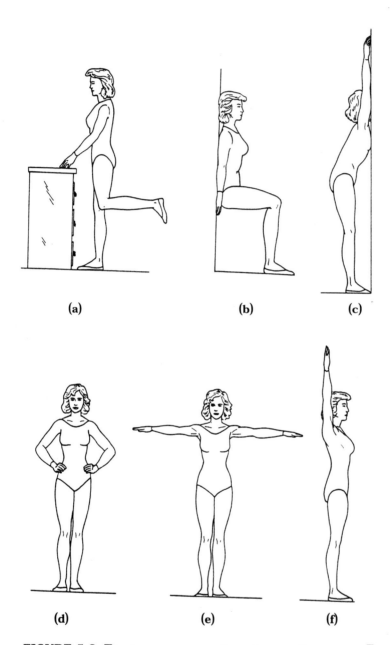

(a)   (b)   (c)

(d)   (e)   (f)

FIGURE 5.3 The home program for osteoporotic women: For strength, flexibility, and position control.

Note: From *Osteoporosis: A guide to prevention and treatment* (pp. 147–155), by J. Aloia, 1989, Champaign, IL: Leisure Press. Copyright 1989 by Leisure Press. Reprinted with permission.

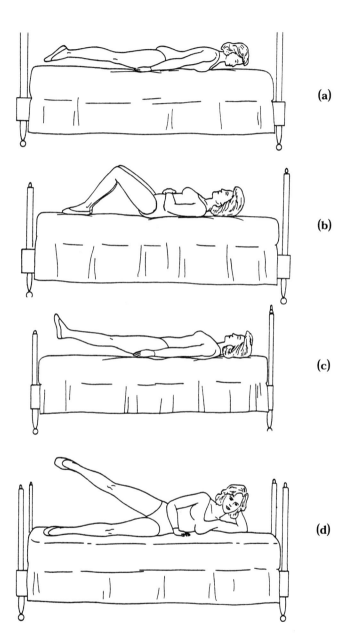

(a)

(b)

(c)

(d)

FIGURE 5.4 The home program for osteoporotic women: For strength, flexibility, and position control—bed exercises.

Note: From *Osteoporosis: A guide to prevention and treatment* (pp. 147–155), by J. Aloia, 1989, Champaign, IL: Leisure Press. Copyright 1989 by Leisure Press. Reprinted with permission.

REFERENCES

Allen, S. (1994). Exercise considerations for postmenopausal women with osteoporosis. *Rheumatology, 7,* 205–214.

Aloia, J. (1989). Exercising for skeletal health. In *Osteoporosis: A guide to prevention and treatment* (pp. 147–155). Champaign, IL: Leisure Press.

Aloia, J., Cohn, S., Ostuni, J., Cane, F., & Ellis, K. (1978). Prevention of involutional bone loss by exercise. *Annals of Internal Medicine, 89,* 356–358.

Aloia, J., Vaswani, A., Yeh, J., & Cohn, S. (1988). Premenopausal bone mass is related to physical activity. *Archives of Internal Medicine, 148,* 121–123.

Aniansson, A., & Gustavson, E. (1981). Physical training in elderly men with specific reference to quadriceps muscle strength and morphology. *Clinical Physiology, 1,* 87–98.

Ayalon, J., Simkin, A., Leichter, I., & Raifmann, S. (1987). Dynamic bone loading exercises for postmenopausal women: Effect on the density of the distal radius. *Archives of Physical Medicine and Rehabilitation, 68,* 280–283.

Bartelink, D. (1957). The role of abdominal pressure in relieving the pressure on the lumbar intervertebral discs. *Journal of Bone and Joint Surgery, 39B,* 718–725.

Blair, S., Gibbons, L., Painter, P., Pate, R., Taylor, C., & Will, J. (1991). *Guidelines for exercise testing and prescription* (4th ed.). Philadelphia: Lea and Febiger.

Brown, A., McCartnet, N., & Sale, D. (1990). Positive adaptations to weight training in the elderly. *Journal of Applied Physiology, 69,* 1725–1733.

Charette, S. L., McEvoy, L., Pyka, G., Snow-Harter, C., Guido, D., Wiswell, R. A., & Marcus, R. (1991). Muscle hypertrophy response to resistance training in older women. *Journal of Applied Physiology, 70,* 1912–1916.

Chestnut, C. (1993). Bone mass and exercise. *American Journal of Medicine, 95* (Suppl. 5A), 34S–36S.

Claus-Walker, J., & Halstead, L. (1982). Metabolic and endocrine changes in spinal cord injury: Compounded neurologic dysfunctions. *Archives of Physical Medicine and Rehabilitation, 63,* 632–638.

Dalsky, G. P., Stocke, K. S., Ehsani, A. A., Slatopolsky, E., Lee, W. C., & Birge, S. J., Jr. (1988). Weight-bearing exercise training and lumbar bone mineral content in postmenopausal women. *Annals of Internal Medicine, 108,* 824–828.

Doyle, F., Brown, J., & LaChance, C. (1970). Relation between bone mass and muscle weight. *Lancet, 1,* 391–393.

Drinkwater, B. L. (1993). Exercise and the prevention of osteoporosis. *Osteoporosis International, 3*(Suppl. 1), 169–171.

Drinkwater, B. L., Nilson, K., Chestnut, C. H. III, Bremner, W. J., Shainholtz, S., & Southworth, M. B. (1984). Bone mineral content of amennorheic and eumenorrheic athletes. *New England Journal of Medicine, 311,* 277–281.

Frontera, W., & Meredith, C. (1989). Strength training in the elderly. In R. Harris & S. Harris (Eds.), *Physical activity, aging, and sports* (pp. 319–331). Albany, NY: Center for the Study of Aging.

Frontera, W., Meredith, C., O'Reilly, K., & Evans, W. (1988). Strength conditioning in older men: Skeletal muscle hypertrophy and improved function. *Journal of Applied Physiology, 64,* 1038–1044.

Geusens, P., & Dequeker, J. (1993). Influence of exercise on bone mineral content and density. *Rheumatology, 14,* 61–70.

Gilsanz, V., Gibbons, D., Carlson, M., Boechat, M., Cann, C., & Schultz, E. (1988). Peak trabecular vertebral density: A comparison of adolescent and adult females. *Calcified Tissue International, 43,* 260–262.

Gutin, B., & Kasper, M. (1992). Can vigorous exercise play a role in osteoporosis prevention? A review. *Osteoporosis International, 2,* 55–69.

Halioua, L., & Anderson, J. (1989). Lifetime calcium intake and physical activity habits: Independent combined effects on the radial bone of healthy premenopausal Caucasian women. *American Journal of Clinical Nutrition, 49,* 534–541.

Halle, J., Schmidt, G., O'Dwyer, K., & Lin, S. (1990). Relationship between trunk muscle torque and bone mineral content of the lumbar spine and hip in healthy postmenopausal women. *Physical Therapy, 70,* 690–699.

Hetland, M., Haarbo, J., & Christensen, C. (1993). Running induces menstrual disturbances but bone mass is unaffected, except in amenorrheic women. *American Journal of Medicine, 95,* 53–60.

Hui, S. L., Slemenda, C. W., & Johnston, C. C. (1990). The contribution of bone loss to postmenopausal osteoporosis. *Osteoporosis International, 1,* 30–34.

Johnston, C., Miller, J., Slemenda, C., Reister, T., Hui, S., Christian, J., & Peacock, M. (1992). Calcium supplementation and increases in bone mineral density in children. *New England Journal of Medicine, 327,* 82–87.

Kritz-Silverstein, D., & Barrett, E. (1994). Grip strength and bone mineral density in older women. *Journal of Bone and Mineral Research, 9,* 45–51.

Krolner, B., & Toft, B. (1983). Vertebral bone loss: An unheeded side effect of therapeutic bed rest. *Clinical Science, 64,* 537–540.

LeBlanc, A., Schneider, V., Krebs, J., Evans, H., Jhingran, S., & Johnson, P. (1987). Spinal bone mineral after 5 weeks of bed rest. *Calcified Tissue International, 41,* 259–261.

Mack, P., LaChance, P., Vose, G., & Vogt, F. (1967). Bone demineralization of foot and hand of Gemini Titan IV, V, and VII astronauts during orbital flight. *American Journal of Roentgenology Radium Therapy and Nuclear Medicine, 100,* 503–511.

Marcus, R. (1992). Secondary forms of osteoporosis. In F. Coe & M. Favus (Eds.), *Disorders of bone and mineral metabolism* (pp. 889–904). New York: Raven Press.

Martin, D., & Novelovitz, M. (1993). Effects of aerobic training on bone mineral density of postmenopausal women. *Journal of Bone Mineral Research, 8,* 931–936.

Matkovic, V., Kostial, K., Simonovic, I., Buzina, R., Brodarec, A., & Nordin, B. (1979). Bone status and fracture rates in two regions of Yugoslavia. *American Journal of Clinical Nutrition, 32,* 540–549.

Menkes, A., Mazel, S., Redmond, R. A., Koffler, K., Libanati, C. R., Gundberg, C. M., Zizic, T. M., Hagberg, J. M., Pratley, R. E., & Hurley, B. F. (1993). Strength training increases regional bone mineral density and bone remodeling in middle-aged and older men. *Journal of Applied Physiology, 74,* 2478–2484.

Nelson, M., Meredith, C., Dawson-Hughes, B., & Evans, W. (1988). Hormone and bone mineral status in endurance trained and sedentary postmenopausal women. *Journal of Clinical Endocrinology and Metabolism, 66,* 927–933.

Nelson, M. E., Fisher, E. C., Dilmanian, F. A., Dallal, G. E., & Evans, W. J. (1991). A 1-year walking program and increased dietary calcium in postmenopausal women: Effects on bone. *American Journal of Clinical Nutrition, 53,* 1304–1311.

Nilsson, B., & Westlin, N. (1971). Bone density in athletes. *Clinical Orthopaedics & Related Research, 77,* 179–182.

Oyster, N., Morton, M., & Linnell, S. (1984). Physical activity and osteoporosis in postmenopausal women. *Medicine and Science in Sports and Exercise, 16,* 44–50.

Pead, M., Skerry, L., & Lanyon, L. (1988). Direct transformation from quiescence to bone formation in the adult periosteum following a single brief period of bone loading. *Journal of Bone Mineral Research, 9,* 97–97.

Pocock, N., Eisman, J., Gwinn, T., Sambrook, P., Kelly P., Freund, J., & Yeates, M. (1989). Muscle strength, physical fitness, and weight but not age predict femoral neck bone mass. *Journal of Bone and Mineral Research, 4,* 441–448.

Pogrund, H., Bloom, R., & Weinberg, H. (1986). Relationship of psoas width to osteoporosis. *Acta Orthopaedica Scandinavica, 57,* 208–210.

Prince, R. L., Smith, M., Dick, I. M., Price, R. I., Webb, P. G., Henderson, N. K., & Harris, M. M. (1991). Prevention of postmenopausal osteoporosis: A comparative study of exercise, calcium supplementation, and hormone replacement therapy. *New England Journal of Medicine, 325,* 1189–1195.

Pyka, G., Lindberger, E., Charette, S., & Marcus, R. (1994). Muscle strength and fiber adaptations to a year-long resistance training program in elderly men and women. *Journal of Gerontology, 49,* M22–M27.

Recker, R. R. (1992). Embryology, anatomy, and microstructure of bone. In F. L. Coe & M. J. Favus (Eds.), *Disorders of bone and mineral metabolism* (pp. 143–221). New York: Raven Press.

Rock, J., & Fortney, S. (1984). Medical and surgical considerations for women in space flight. *Obstetrical and Gynecological Survey, 39,* 525–535.

Rogers, M. A., & Evans, W. J. (1993). Changes in skeletal muscle with aging: Effects of exercise training. *Exercise & Sports Sciences Review, 21,* 65–102.

Rubin, C., & Lanyon, L. (1984). Regulation of bone formation by applied dynamic loads. *Journal of Bone and Joint Surgery, 66A,* 397–402.

Rubin, C., & Lanyon, L. (1985). Regulation of bone mass by mechanical strain magnitude. *Calcified Tissue International, 37,* 411–417.

Sandler, R. B., Slemenda, C. W., LaPorte, R. E., Cauley, J. A., Schramm, M. M., Barresi, M. L., & Kriska, A. M. (1985). Postmenopausal bone density and milk consumption in childhood and adolescence. *American Journal of Clinical Nutrition, 42,* 270–274.

Schneider, V., & McDonald, J. (1984). Skeletal calcium homeostasis and counter-measures to prevent disuse osteoporosis. *Calcified Tissue International, 36,* s151–s154.

Sinaki, M. (1982). Postmenopausal spinal osteoporosis physical therapy and rehabilitation principles. *Mayo Clinic Proceedings, 57,* 699–703.

Sinaki, M. (1989). Exercise and osteoporosis. *Archives of Physical Medicine and Rehabilitation, 70,* 220–229.

Sinaki, M., & Mikkelsen, B. (1984). Postmenopausal spinal osteoporosis, flexion versus extension exercises. *Archives of Physical and Medical Rehabilitation, 65,* 593–596.

Sinaki, M., & Offord, K. (1988). Physical activity in postmenopausal women: Effect on back muscle strength and bone mineral density of the spine. *Archives of Physical Medicine and Rehabilitation, 69,* 277–280.

Slemenda, C., Christian, J., Williams, C., Norton, J., & Johnston, C. (1991). Genetic determinants of bone mass in adult women: A reevaluation of the twin model and potential importance of gene interaction on heritability estimates. *Journal of Bone and Mineral Research, 6,* 561–567.

Slemenda, C., Miller, J., Hui, S., Reister, T., & Johnston, C. (1991). Role of physical activity in the development of skeletal bone mass in children. *Journal of Bone and Mineral Research, 6,* 1227–1233.

Stevenson, J., Lees, B., Davenport, M., Cust, M., & Ganger, K. (1989). Determinants of bone density in normal women: Risk factors for future osteoporosis? *British Medical Journal, 298,* 924–928.

Turner, C., Forwood, M., Rho, J., & Yoshikawa, T. (1994). Mechanical loading thresholds for lamellar and woven bone formation. *Journal of Bone Mineral Research, 9,* 87–97.

Uhthoff, H., & Jaworski, Z. (1978). Bone loss in response to long-term immobilization. *Journal of Bone and Joint Surgery, 60B,* 420–429.

Westlin, N. (1974). Loss of bone mineral after Colles' fracture. *Clinical Orthopedics and Related Research, 20,* 194–199.

Wolman, R., Clark, P., McNally, E., Harries, M., & Reeve, J. (1990). Menstrual state and exercise as determinants of spinal trabecular bone density in female athletes. *British Journal of Medicine, 301,* 516–518.

Young, D., Niklowits, W., Brown, R., & Jee, W. (1986). Immobilization-associated osteoporosis in primates. *Bone, 7,* 109–117.

Zhang, H., Feldbaum, P., & Fortney, J. (1992). Moderate physical activity and bone density among perimenopausal women. *Journal of Public Health, 82,* 736–738.

Zimmerman, C., Schmidt, G., Brooks, J., Kinsey, W., & Eekhoff, Y. (1990). Relationship of extremity muscle torque and bone mineral density in postmenopausal women. *Physical Therapy, 70,* 302–309.

6

Bone Remodeling and the Development of Osteoporosis

M. Susan Burke

Two to ten percent of the skeleton is remodeled yearly, in a process that takes three to five months to complete.

—H. Fleisch

Along with genetic and other factors, peak bone mass is augmented by adequate calcium, vitamin D, exercise, and a generally healthy lifestyle. These measures help achieve and maintain as high a bone mass as possible and are vital complements for optimum bone health. In the ideal world, one would prefer to prevent osteoporosis from ever developing. However, the dwindling estrogen contribution to the remodeling sequence at the time of menopause results in at least some bone loss. Genetic makeup, other hormones, and certain medications can also negatively influence bone mass. This does not mean, however, that someone is doomed to develop osteoporosis. Pharmaceutical agents to help maintain bone mass after menopause, when bone loss can be particularly rapid, are now available. In order to appreciate how specific therapies act to prevent or treat osteoporosis, the process of bone remodeling and how it can lead to bone loss will be reviewed.

BONE REMODELING AND THE DEVELOPMENT OF OSTEOPOROSIS

Patients often have trouble understanding that their bones become weaker and more porous with age. It is difficult for them to imagine that their bones are deteriorating inside them when archeologists can unearth well-preserved bones that are thousands of years old. Although maximum height is achieved in late adolescence, the structure of bone continues to be renovated and remodeled. This can be compared to a house, which, once built, benefits from continued maintenance. New bone replaces old bone in a closely linked process called the bone remodeling sequence. Remodeling helps the bone maintain its structural integrity while also serving as an ion reservoir for calcium homeostasis. Two to 10% of the skeleton is remodeled yearly (Fleisch, 1997), and the process takes from 3 to 5 months to complete.

The skeleton is comprised of 80% cortical (compact) bone, located mostly on outer surfaces; the remainder is inner trabecular (cancellous or spongy) bone, which predominates in the vertebrae, proximal femur, and distal radius. If less new bone is formed to replace the old bone that is dissolved away, a net loss of bone occurs. Structurally, this fragile bone is more likely to break with less trauma—the hallmark of osteoporosis. Although remodeling occurs in both types of bone, 80% occurs in trabecular bone. This explains why fractures in regions of high trabecular content—spine, hip, and wrist—are such common sequelae of this disease.

Bone Resorption

In this remodeling sequence, bone cells lie quiescent until osteoclasts (bone resorbing cells) are stimulated to resorb a small area of bone. Osteoclast activity is increased by factors such as parathyroid hormone (PTH), vitamin D, and thyroxine and decreased by estrogen, testosterone, calcitonin, and even cytokines from osteoblasts (bone forming cells). Local factors, such as prostaglandins and interleukins, may also exert either a stimulatory or inhibitory effect. Calcium homeostasis is integrally tied to this process (see

Table 6.1). A low calcium level stimulates the secretion of PTH. This activates the osteoclasts to release lysosomal enzymes, which digest bone matrix, causing the release of calcium and other bone minerals. Collagen and noncollagen proteins such as hydroxyproline, pyridinoline, and deoxypyridinoline are also released.

CLINICAL CORRELATION

Many older women are found to have higher than normal levels of PTH (secondary hyperparathyroidism) because of low calcium intake and an age-related decrease in vitamin D production. Calcium supplementation may normalize PTH levels in some patients.

TABLE 6.1   Bone Remodeling and Its Clinical Correlations

Phase of remodeling sequence	Quiescence	Bone resorption by osteoclasts	Reversal	Bone formation by osteoclasts	Quiescence

Stimulating factors		Parathyroid hormone Vitamin D Thyroxine	Growth hormones Parathyroid hormone Estrogen Testosterone Cytokines Prostaglandins Vitamin D
Inhibiting factors		Estrogen Calcitonin Testosterone Alendronate Raloxifene	Corticosteroids Alcohol Smoking
Markers		Urinary hydroxyproline Pyridinoline cross-links (pyridinoline and deoxypyridinoline)	Bone-specific alkaline phosphatase Serum osteocalcin

Urine levels of pyridinoline (Pyrilinks-D) and deoxypyridinoline (Osteomark N-Tx) can be used clinically to evaluate how much bone is being resorbed at any one time, and possibly to monitor the impact of drug treatment on this process. Hydroxyproline can also be measured, but is less specific.

Most therapeutic modalities that are presently available act by inhibiting osteoclast action on bone resorption. This results in a reduced cavity size, while allowing bone formation to continue.

Reversal

The transition from resorption to formation is called reversal (Rodan, 1996). After the resorption cavity is formed, a cement line is laid down by macrophage-type mononuclear cells, limiting further resorption of bone in that area. The cement line is rich in osteopontin, which may serve to shut off osteoclast activity and stimulate osteoblast activity.

Bone Formation

Through the action of local factors, such as insulin-like growth factors and osteopontin, and systemic factors like PTH, vitamin D (the latter two under investigation as therapeutic agents), estrogen, testosterone, and calcitonin, osteoblasts are recruited to the resorbed cavity (Baron, 1996). First, these cells secrete the osseous organic matrix. Later, calcium and phosphorus become incorporated into the lattice-like organic framework. Adequate calcium intake is necessary for proper mineralization.

CLINICAL CORRELATION

The osteoblast's membrane contains abundant amounts of alkaline phosphatase, and a serum measurement of this bone-specific alkaline phosphatase can be used as a marker of bone formation. Another such marker is osteocalcin, released by osteoblasts as they lay down new bone.

Development of Osteoporosis

Generally, the cavity formed by bone resorption and the matrix deposited during bone formation are approximately equal. These processes are linked together, perhaps by bone formation factors released during bone resorption (Rodan, 1996). Any factor that influences bone resorption and formation can affect this balance. In postmenopausal osteoporosis, the loss of estrogen's inhibitory effect on resorption and its stimulatory effect on formation leads to an imbalance and net loss of bone. No treatment presently available can restore areas of bone that have been completely resorbed. Although it is preferable to prevent significant bone loss from occurring in the first place, many therapeutic agents can strengthen the remaining bone structure and decrease fracture risk.

REFERENCES

Baron, R. (1996). Anatomy and ultrastructure of bone. In M. J. Favus (Ed.), *Primer on the metabolic bone diseases and disorders of mineral metabolism* (3rd ed., p. 15). Philadelphia: Lippincott-Raven.

Rodan, G. (1996). Coupling of bone resorption and formation during bone remodeling. In R. Marcus, D. Feldman, & J. Kelsey (Eds.), *Osteoporosis* (p. 290). New York: Academic Press.

7

Osteoporosis: Patient Identification and Evaluation

Ellen Field-Munves

> With osteoporosis reaching epidemic proportions, women
> are becoming more aware of their individual bone mass
> measurements.
>
> —E. F. Munves

EPIDEMIOLOGY AND PREVALENCE

Approximately 23 million postmenopausal women, age 50 and older, have low bone mass. Of these, 8.1 million women have established osteoporosis, with bone mass measurements equal to or below 2.5 standard deviations from the mean bone mass of young normals, utilizing the criteria established by the World Health Organization. The National Osteoporosis Foundation has estimated that in the next 20 years there will be 80 million postmenopausal women, with potentially one out of every two White women experiencing a fracture due to osteoporosis in her lifetime (Ross, Davis, Epstein, & Wasnich, 1991). The estimated lifetime fracture risk for women age 50 is 40% (Kanis, 1994, pp. 1–6). Specifically, percent risk for fracture at proximal femur, vertebrae, or distal forearm, is 17.5%, 15.6%, and 16%, respectively. The vertebral fractures include only those that are clinically diagnosed (Kanis, 1994, pp. 1–6).

With one vertebral fracture at baseline, there is a five-fold increase in vertebral fracture (Ross et al., 1991). Two or more vertebral fractures at baseline hold a 12-fold increase in vertebral fracture. One symptomatic vertebral fracture at baseline increases hip fracture risk two-fold (Kanis, 1994, p. 8). The effect of a one standard deviation in baseline lumbar spine bone mineral density is comparable to the effect of a 17-year increase in age on the risk of a vertebral fracture (Melton, Atkinson, O'Fallon, Wahner, & Riggs, 1993). The effect of a one standard deviation bone mineral density of the femoral neck or femoral trochanter is comparable to a 14- or 13-year increase in age, respectively, on the risk of an incident hip fracture.

The prevalence of osteoporotic hip fracture in the United States is 300,000 fractures annually (U.S. Congress, 1994), with an excess of 24% mortality in the first year (Ray, Chan, Thamer, & Melton, 1997). Note that 50% of those who sustain hip fractures never fully recover (Consensus Development Conference, 1993), and 25% require long-term nursing home care. The lifetime risk of death associated with an osteoporotic hip fracture is comparable to that of breast cancer (Cummings, Black, & Rubin, 1989), and death from complications of osteoporosis is greater than the risk of death from breast cancer and uterine cancer combined (Hawker, 1996).

The economic burden of osteoporotic fracture in utilization of health care dollars is immense. In 1995, 3.4 million outpatient physician, outpatient hospital, and emergency room visits were due to osteoporotic fracture. Approximately 2.2 million home health care visits were due to osteoporotic fracture, with almost 60% due to hip fracture alone (Ray et al., 1997). There were 432,448 hospitalizations for osteoporotic fracture for persons aged 45 or older in 1995, with 57% for hip fractures, 6.8% for spinal fractures, 3.1% for forearm fractures, and 33% for fractures at other sites (Ray et al., 1997). There were 179,221 nursing home stays, 76.9% due to hip fractures (Ray et al., 1997). Estimated health care costs for that year were almost $14 billion (Compston, Cooper, & Kanis, 1995). The rate of hip fractures is expected to increase multifold due to the growing senior population.

In order to prevent morbidity and/or mortality from osteoporosis, one needs to consider and implement early intervention, including medication when necessary, and routine use of calcium, vitamin D, and exercise. To utilize early intervention, one must be able to have early diagnosis. This is the key to prevention of future outcomes in patients with low bone mass.

Vertebral fractures may cause height loss, kyphosis, and back pain, impacting on quality of life as well as survival. Multiple thoracic compression fractures may cause restrictive lung disease, and multiple lumbar compression fractures may lead to abdominal distention, pain, anorexia, and early satiety. Certainly, the psychological impact of this disease is not to be overlooked, as patients may suffer from loss of self-esteem, depression, fear of falling, fear of subsequent fracture, and loss of independence, as well as an increase in morbidity and mortality.

DIAGNOSIS

Osteoporosis is defined as low bone mass with irreversible microarchitectural changes which can lead to an increased risk for fragility fractures. In normal bone, there are remodeling processes that account for a steady-state balance of osteoclastic (bone resorption) and osteoblastic (bone formation) activity (see Figure 7.1). The shift of increase in bone resorption over bone formation may account for net loss in bone mass and increase risk for fracture in osteoporotic patients. Increased rates of bone turnover may be measured by markers of resorption and formation, which include urinary calcium excretion, free pyridinoline, N-telopeptide of collagen, osteocalcin, bone

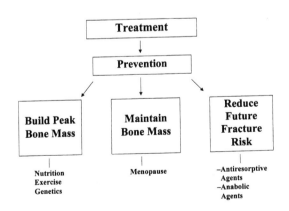

FIGURE 7.1   Recent approaches to the management of osteoporosis.

specific alkaline phosphatase, and carboxy-terminal propeptide of type I procollagen. (For more specific details, see chapter 6.)

Current availability of bone densitometry has been quite useful in clinical practice to diagnose low bone mass, predict risk for future fracture, and monitor effects of therapeutic interventions (Compston et al., 1995). Most experts agree that dual-energy x-ray absorptiometry (DXA) is the gold standard, both for fracture risk assessment and monitoring effects of treatment. Clinical risk factors may be poor predictors of low bone mass and risk for fracture (Slemenda, Hui, & Longcope, 1990). In recent years, there has been tremendous growth in the number of peripheral and central bone densitometers, as well as entrance of quantitative ultrasound measurement into the marketplace.

X-ray techniques to measure bone density date back to 1939 (Mack, O'Brien, Smith, & Bauman, 1939). Cameron and Sorensen described the technique of single photon absorptiometry (SPA) in 1963 (Cameron & Sorenson, 1963). This technique utilizes iodine 125 (^{125}I) to generate photon energy. Bone mineral content is quantified in the region of interest, by comparing the amount of attenuation of the photon beam with attenuation by standards created from ashed bone. This technique can only be used in areas such as the forearm or os calcis (heel), which are not surrounded by soft tissue masses. This method is accurate as well as precise. Dual photon absorptiometry (DPA) uses gadolinium 153 (153 Gd), which allows for measurement of bone density in spine and proximal femur, which are surrounded by large soft tissue masses (Dunn, Wahner, & Riggs, 1980; Wahner et al., 1983). Although accurate, DPA is not precise enough to allow for monitoring changes in bone mass over time. DXA has been approved since 1988. DXA uses an x-ray tube instead of 153 Gd, which decreases scan time and x-ray exposure (Lees & Stevenson, 1992; Kelly, Slovik, Schoenfeld, & Neer, 1988; Povilles, Tremollieres, Todorovsky, & Ribot, 1991). Precision of DXA is superior to that of DPA. Most DXA scanners are pencil-beam rectilinear scanners; however, newer technology called fan-beam decreases scan times further.

Quantitative computed tomography (QCT) measurements of bone density are three-dimensional volumetric measurements of vertebral body trabecular bone (Genant, Cann, Ettinger, & Gordan, 1982; Cann, 1987; Genant, Block, Steiger, & Gluer, 1987). Skin radiation doses are higher in QCT, but the overall significant dose is small since only a small area is being irradiated. This dose is higher than with DPA or pencil beam DXA (Kalender, 1992).

The ability of a single bone density measurement to predict fracture risk has been demonstrated in many prospective trials (Wasnich, Ross, Heilbrun, & Vogel, 1985; Hui, Slemenda, & Johnston, 1988; Gardsell, Johnell, & Nilsson, 1991; Cummings et al., 1993; Mazess, Barden, Ettinger, & Schulz, 1988). Even though bone mass measurements at different skeletal sites (e.g., lumbar spine, hip, radius, and os calcis) are predictive of fracture risk, better prediction is made using site-specific prediction, particularly at the hip (Melton et al., 1993). Global fracture risk predicts risk of any type of osteoporotic fracture, whereas site-specific fracture risk predicts risk of specific types of fracture, such as spine or hip fracture.

BMD INTERPRETATION

The computer printout of bone mineral density includes an image of the skeletal site measured, bone mineral density in grams per centimeter squared, bone mineral content in grams, and the area of the region in centimeters squared. Two values, the T-score and the Z-score, are reported. The T-score is expressed as the number of standard deviations that the patient bone mineral density is away from the mean of young normals and is the value that defines the treatment threshold. Typically, 1 SD is equal to a 10% to 12% difference in bone mineral density. The Z-score is the comparison of the patient bone mineral density to age and sex-matched cohorts. It is also expressed as the number of standard deviations away from the reference population. The Z-score may be helpful to determine which patients have osteoporosis out of proportion to others of the same age, and in whom a secondary work up is indicated. T-scores and Z-scores are standard scores not unique to bone mineral density testing. Bone mass declines with age. The mechanisms contributing to this decline are elaborated on in chapter 6.

Bone mineral density is the most accurate predictor of fracture risk (Consensus Development Conference, 1993; Compston et al., 1995). The ability of bone mass measurement to predict fracture risk is stronger than the association between systolic blood pressure and stroke-associated mortality, and between serum cholesterol and coronary artery events (Compston et al., Kanis, 1994, pp. 1–20). The risk of fracture increases approximately two-fold in the vertebral spine and approximately three-fold in the femoral neck for each standard deviation decline in bone density (Cummings et al., 1993). The World Health Organization (WHO) defines normal bone mass as a T-score above −1, low bone mass or osteopenia as a T-score between −1 and −2.5, and osteoporosis is a T-score at or below −2.5. Patients with fracture *in addition* to T-scores −2.5 or below are classified as having "severe or established" osteoporosis. These criteria were intended as diagnostic criteria, not thresholds for therapeutic interventions, which may depend on other criteria than bone density, such as prior fractures, age, family history of fracture, and other risk factors. Note that there are currently several medications which have been approved by the United States Federal Drug Administration for the prevention and treatment of osteoporosis. These medications will be discussed in the following chapter.

There is a summary of available bone mass measurement technologies capable of predicting risk for fracture (Hans et al., 1996; Black et al., 1992). These technologies measure bone mass at several sites including spine, hip, forearm, finger, heel, shin, and total body (see Table 7.1).

Fracture risk may be global or site-specific. Global fracture risk may be assessed at different skeletal sites (Melton et al., 1993). For example, the

TABLE 7.1 B.M.D. Technologies*

Method	Body site	Effective radiation dose*
DXA Dual—energy x-ray absorptiometry	Hip Spine Total body	Significantly less than standard chest x-ray

p DXA
    Peripheral dual—energy x-ray
    absorptiometry
	Forearm
	Finger
	Heel
		Significantly less than standard chest x-ray

SXA
    Single—energy x-ray
    Absorptiometry
	Heel	Significantly less than standard chest x-ray

QUS Quantitative ultrasound	Heel Shin	None

QCT
    Quantitative computed
    tomography
	Spine	Less than or equal to standard chest x-ray

pQCT
    Peripheral quantitative
    computed tomography
	Forearm	Significantly less than standard chest x-ray

*Note—effective radiation dose is equal to radiation that reaches internal organs.

Note: From Jergas, M., & Genant, H. K. (1993). Current methods and recent advances in the diagnosis of osteoporosis. *Arthritis and Rheumatism, 36,* 1649–1662.

spine and femoral neck appear to be reasonable predictors of global fracture risk. In elderly patients, the 33% radial site can predict nonspine fracture risk (Hui et al., 1989). Proximal femur sites are excellent predictors of site-specific hip fracture (Cummings et al., 1993). It is difficult to determine which site is best able to predict site-specific spine fracture risk. In patients age 65 years or older, vertebral bone mineral density may be falsely elevated due to osteoarthritis and facet joint sclerosis, or aortic calcification (Drinka, DeSmet, Bauwens, & Rogot, 1992; Frye et al., 1992). In elderly patients, bone mass in different regions of the skeleton appears to be concordant (Povilles, Tremollieres, & Ribot, 1993; Arlot, Sornay-Rendu, Garnero, Vey-Marty, & Delmas, 1997; Nelson, Molley, & Kleerekoper, 1998). However, if the spine is the only site measured in older patients, and arthritis or aortic calcification are present, diagnosis of osteoporosis may be missed (Greenspan, Maitland-Ramsey, & Myers, 1996). In patients age 65 years or older, the hip, wrist, heel, finger, or forearm may be more accurate sites than the spine for the diagnosis of osteoporosis (Povilles et al., 1993; Arlot et al., 1997; Nelson et al., 1998). In younger patients, the anteroposterior spine is most often used to predict risk of spine fracture. It is more common to have discordant bone loss in younger individuals, meaning that a given patient may be normal at one site, but have low bone mass at another (Povilles et al., 1993). The site chosen for evaluation is important in making the appropriate diagnosis as noted previously. The proximal femur appears less likely to be affected by age-related skeletal abnormalities, and is also less likely to be normal in the face of low spine density than the converse. Additionally, proximal femur fractures have the greatest risk for comorbidity and mortality. Therefore, if only one site could be measured, the proximal femur would be the preferred choice.

Central bone mineral density measurements on a serial basis may be a reliable means to monitor therapy. However, it is generally accepted that significant changes in bone mineral density due to therapy may require two years for spine and three years or more for proximal femur. Monitoring may improve long-term patient compliance and perhaps detect nonresponders. Note that increases in bone mineral density may not accurately reflect reduction in fracture risk (Cummings, Black, & Vogt, 1996). It may take at least two years or more to determine if a patient has responded to therapy on the basis of bone mineral density changes with currently accepted therapeutic options (Nguyen, Sambrook, & Eisman, 1997). However, more frequent monitoring of bone mineral density is justified in patients on corticosteroids at moderate or high doses, particularly in view of more rapid bone loss, seen especially in the first three to six months of therapy (Saag et al., 1998).

PERIPHERAL BMD TECHNOLOGY

We have multiple choices in available devices for measurement of bone density. Newer, lower cost, and portable peripheral technology has entered the marketplace, opening up opportunities for the physician to study larger populations of patients. With the National Osteoporosis Foundation estimate of 80 million postmenopausal women in the next 20 years, it would seem appropriate to utilize these less expensive and more portable studies. However, single-site measurements present challenges both in discordance of bone mass between skeletal sites as well as their ability to monitor serial changes in bone mineral density (Povilles et al., 1993; Arlot et al., 1997; Blake, Patel, & Fogelman, 1998; Miller & McClung, 1996; Miller et al., 1998).

In peripheral bone mass measurement using the WHO criteria for diagnosis of low bone mass, the potential of misdiagnoses may be lessened by accepting a therapeutic threshold at a T-score −1.0 or greater. By utilizing this score, accuracy errors of the individual technologies would be minimized (Miller et al., 1998; Ross et al., 1995; Cummings et al., 1990; Yates, Ross, Lydick, & Epstein, 1995; Wasnich, 1993). Ultimately, therapeutic intervention at this T-score threshold may have the best opportunity for reducing lifetime fracture risk (Miller et al., 1998). However, because bone loss at single-site measurements may be discordant, additional guidelines have been suggested for perimenopausal patients with normal peripheral measurements (Miller et al., 1998). Additionally, guidelines have been suggested for postmenopausal women identified as having low bone mass by peripheral bone mass measurements (see Table 7.2). These women may not need central bone mass measurements (Miller et al., 1998) (see Table 7.3).

Quantitative ultrasound (QUS) is a technique that measures bone mass and strength and estimates bone microarchitecture (Langton, Evans, Hodgskinson, & Riggs, 1990; Evans & Tavakoli, 1990; Tavakoli & Evans, 1991; Gluer et al., 1992). It detects the transmission of high-frequency sound waves across bone and measures both broadband ultrasound attenuation (BUA) and the speed of sound (SOS) in bone, both of which are higher in normal bone than osteoporotic bone (Langton et al., 1990; Evans & Tavakoli,

TABLE 7.2 Patients with Normal Screening Peripheral BMD Who Should Receive a Central Bone Mass Measurement

- Postmenopausal patients not on estrogen replacement therapy (ERT) concerned about osteoporosis, and concerned about prevention, who would consider ERT, bisphosphonates, or selective estrogen receptor modulators (SERMs) if a low bone mass is discovered.
- Maternal history of hip fracture, smoking, tall (> 5' 7") or thin (< 125 lbs.)
- Patients on medications associated with bone loss (steroids, gonadotropin—releasing hormone (G R H) agonists, and antiseizure medication, etc.)
- Patients with secondary conditions associated with low bone mass (hyperthyroidism, post transplantation, malabsorption, hemigastrectomy, hyperparathyroidism, prolactinoma, immobilization, and so forth.
- Patients who have high urinary collagen cross links N-telopeptide [NTX], C-telopeptide [CTx], and deoxypyridinoline [DpD]), i.e., 1.0 standard deviation or more above the upper limit for the premenopausal range, who therefore, may be rapid bone losers.
- History of fragility fractures.

Note: From Miller et al. (1998). The challenges of peripheral bone density: Which patients need additional central density skeletal measurements? *American Journal of Medical Science, 1,* 211–217.

1990; Tavakoli & Evans, 1991; Gluer et al., 1992). The reports give a ratio of BUA to SOS, known as either the quantitative ultrasound index (Q. I) or stiffness index (SI). Body sites measured include heal and shin, and there is no ionizing radiation exposure. QUS is an effective method for predicting fracture risk (Hans et al., 1996). There is much research into practical applications of ultrasound technology in evaluation of osteoporosis.

TABLE 7.3 Postmenopausal Patients Who May Not Need the Central Skeletal Measurement Once Screen for Low Bone Mass by Peripheral Techniques

- Women starting ERT based on the diagnosis of low bone mass, whose NTx/CTx/DpD are low (lower quartile of premenopausal range) after starting ERT.
- Elderly patients with significant competing risks for reduced life expectancy, yet placed on treatment for osteoporosis to reduce fracture risk.
- Patients with elevated peripheral bone mass (> 1.0 SD) who have no risk factors for low bone mass.
- Patients who have a > 50% reduction from baseline (3 months after starting treatment) in NTx, CTx, or DpD on therapy.

Note: From Miller et al. (1998). The challenges of peripheral bone density: Which patients need additional central density skeletal measurements? *American Journal of Medical Science, 1,* 211–217.

IDENTIFICATION OF PATIENTS AT RISK

Who should be evaluated? Generally it is agreed that all postmenopausal women with increased risk for fracture should be considered for bone mass testing. The National Osteoporosis Foundation has included risk factors for osteoporotic fracture in their recently published guidelines. Nonmodifiable factors including personal history of fracture as an adult and history of fracture in a first-degree relative, as well as cigarette smoking and low body weight, have been demonstrated in large prospective studies to be important risk factors for fracture even independent of bone density (National Osteoporosis Foundation, 1998). Basically, the National Osteoporosis Foundation guidelines recommend testing for all women greater or equal to age 65 (independent of risk factors), all postmenopausal women less than 65 years of age, with at least one additional risk factor for osteoporosis other than menopause (see Table 7.4), all postmenopausal women who present with fractures, all women considering therapy for osteoporosis and for whom

TABLE 7.4 Risk Factors for Osteoporotic Fracture

Nonmodifiable:

- personal history of fracture as an adult
- history of fracture in first-degree relative
- Caucasian race
- advanced age
- female sex
- dementia
- poor health/frailty

Potentially Modifiable:

- current cigarette smoking
- low body weight (< 127 pounds)
- estrogen deficiency:
  early menopause (less than age 45) or bilateral ovariectomy
  prolonged premenopausal amenorrhea (> 1 year)
- low calcium intake (lifelong)
- alcoholism
- impaired eyesight despite adequate correction
- recurrent falls
- inadequate physical activity
- poor health/frailty

BMD test results would influence their decision, and all women who have been receiving hormone replacement therapy for a prolonged period. Some experts have classified common forms of osteoporosis as idiopathic, Type 1, and Type 2 osteoporosis. A variety of secondary causes, including genetic, metabolic, drug-induced, and so on have also been identified.

Type 1 osteoporosis would generally be considered to include postmenopausal women with predominantly rapid trabecular bone loss, with associated increased risk for spinal fractures and distal forearm fractures. Type 2 osteoporosis is found in both men and women, generally past age 70, with associated fractures of femoral neck, proximal forearm, proximal tibia, and pelvis (both cortical and trabecular bone). These patients frequently have high intact PTH (parathyroid hormone). Both groups have decreased mean circulating levels of $1,25\ (OH_2)D$ (vitamin D) (Krane & Holick, 1994).

Disabling and devastating fractures, which are potential outcomes of osteoporosis, may present with pain, which can limit one's daily activities and have other sequelae. Spinal fractures, dorsal or lumbar, may occur after lifting, bending, reaching, etc., and may occur with little trauma. Not infrequently these fractures may be asymptomatic, presenting with height loss or vertebral loss known as dowager's hump. These occur after anterior vertebral collapse, causing a wedge-shaped deformity. Many patients have associated osteoarthritis which may contribute to chronic back pain. Occasionally, patients may complain of "sciatica type" symptoms, but frank spinal cord compression is unlikely. Patients may develop abdominal distention and ileus from kyphotic posture, which may be worsened by use of narcotic analgesic agents. Most osteoporotic spinal fractures occur in the mid- or lower-thoracic vertebral bodies, or upper-lumbar vertebral bodies. In the absence of fracture, standard x-ray imaging is poorly sensitive in detecting early bone loss, as it may take at least a 30% bone loss before x-ray demineralization may be seen.

SECONDARY CAUSES OF OSTEOPOROSIS

It is important to consider other causes of low bone mass, particularly since treatment may be directed at the primary etiology. This could significantly impact the patient's prognosis, particularly in the case of malignancy, for example. There are many publications on secondary causes of osteoporosis, and this author would recommend a review of these publications. A comprehensive list of diseases and drugs associated with increased risk for osteoporosis in adults is outlined in the National Osteoporosis Foundation Physician's Guide to Prevention and Treatment of Osteoporosis (National Osteoporosis Foundation, 1998). A summary of that information is provided in Table 7.5.

Exogenous glucocorticoid excess is the most frequent cause of secondary osteoporosis. Bone loss may be rapid, particularly in children and women over age 50. Endogenous glucocorticoid excess, or Cushing's syndrome, may be due to a curable condition, and treatment may lead to recovery of bone loss. Glucocorticoid induced osteoporosis is due to both decreased bone formation and increased bone resorption. Secondary hyperparathyroidism may be important, particularly early on, leading to rapid bone loss with an associated increase in bone resorption (Lems et al., 1998; Reid, 1997).

Fractures, most commonly vertebral and rib, may occur after prolonged exposure; however, other fractures may occur as well (Reid, 1997). It is reported that fracture incidence in glucocorticoid excess may be between 30% and 50% (Adinoff & Hollister, 1983). Glucocorticoid inhibition of new bone formation may be due to direct effect on bone cells and production of local regulatory factors (Canalis, 1996). Patients may have hypercalciuria due to high rates of resorption, which may account for secondary hyperparathyroidism, despite the fact that elevated PTH levels are not always found.

Glucocorticoids suppress collagen synthesis, with delayed wound healing and thinning of the skin seen in many rheumatoid patients. Twenty-five (OH)D may be normal or slightly decreased and $1,25 (OH_2)D$ is usually normal. Steroids inhibit calcium absorption from the stomach by direct (non-Vitamin D dependent) effect. Withdrawal or decreasing steroids may help slow the process. Adding calcitriol [$1,25 (OH_2)D_3$] in doses of 0.5 to 1.0 mcg per day with 1,000 milligrams of supplemental calcium may prevent the defect in intestinal calcium absorption. Vitamin D metabolites may be effective as well. Certainly, serum and urinary calcium should be monitored. Cushing's syndrome can result in asymptomatic fractures in ribs, pubic, or ischial rami, despite bone loss in the spine. These may heal with excessive callus formation, appearing somewhat like the pseudofractures seen in osteomalacia.

When patients are started on glucocorticoids, they should be monitored with bone density measurements as early as six months, and those patients with low bone mass or fracture should be considered for therapy with antiresorptive agents (Reid, 1997; Adachi et al., 1997; Saag et al., 1998). Even though the primary defect may be on bone formation, bone is also lost by resorption. Doses of 7.5 mg daily of prednisone, or its equivalent,

TABLE 7.5 Diseases and Drugs Associated with an Increased Risk of Generalized Osteoporosis in Adults

Diseases	Drugs
Acromegaly	Aluminum
Adrenal atrophy and Addison's disease	Anticonvulsants
Amyloidosis	Cigarette smoking
Ankylosing spondylitis	Cytotoxic drugs
Chronic obstructive pulmonary disease	Excessive alcohol
Congenital porphyria	Excessive thyroxine
Cushing's syndrome	Glucocorticosteroids adrenocorticotropin
Endometriosis	Gonadotropin releasing hormone
Epidermolysis bullosa	Agonists
Gastrectomy	Heparin
Gonadal insufficiency	Lithium
(Primary and secondary)	Tamoxifen
Hemochromatosis	(Premenopausal use)
Hemophilia	
Hyperparathyroidism	
Hypophosphatasia	
Idiopathic scoliosis	
Insulin-dependent diabetes mellitus	
Lymphoma and leukemia	
Malabsorption syndromes	
Mastocytosis	
Multiple myeloma	
Multiple sclerosis	
Nutritional disorders	
Osteogenesis Imperfecta	
Parenteral nutrition	
Pernicious anemia	
Rheumatoid arthritis	
Sarcoidosis	
Severe liver disease, especially primary biliary cirrhosis	
Thalassemia	
Thyrotoxicosis	
Tumor secretion of parathyroid	
Hormone—related peptide	

have been associated with osteoporosis (Reid, 1997). However, bone loss with lower doses over time, especially in conjunction with additional risk factors, may be seen.

Hypogonadism may be a cause of low bone mass in men and women, distinct from the typical postmenopausal osteoporosis in women and age-related decline in gonadal function in older men. Causes include such diseases as primary hypogonadism, hyperprolactinemia, hemochromatosis, Klinefelter's and Kallmann's syndromes, premature ovarian failure, mumps orchitis, anorexia nervosa, and excessive exercise-induced hypogonadism (Orlic & Raisz, 1999). Receptors for both estrogen and androgen are present in the skeleton (Vanderscheueren & Bouillon, 1995). Although testosterone is generally anabolic since it is aromatized to estradiol, which is antiresorptive, it can be difficult to show discrete actions. Men may develop high turnover bone loss with estrogen deficiency secondary to either receptor defects or aromatase deficiency (Bilezikian, Morishima, Bell, & Grumbach, 1998). Hormone levels should be assessed in appropriate patients; and if deficiencies are found, treatment should be directed as indicated with hormone therapy.

In thyrotoxicosis, one can see increased bone resorption, which may be accompanied by increased excretion of calcium and phosphorus in both urine and feces. There is a compensatory increase in bone formation. PTH and $1,25 (OH_2)D$ are generally low. If the disease is of longer duration, skeletal bone loss may be significant (Leb, Warnkross, & Obermayer-Pietsch, 1994). It is imperative to monitor hypothyroid patients on replacement therapy with serial TSH measurements to rule out oversuppression, because this can cause bone loss. Bone loss has been seen with high dose thyroid hormone used for thyroid cancer patients. These patients should have routine assessment of skeletal status, with appropriate therapeutic interventions as indicated.

In acromegaly, one may have hypercalciuria and net negative calcium balance, with secondary panhypopituitarism and hypogonadism, and potentially low bone mass. There may be increased production of IGF-1, which can cause increased bone remodeling, and then associated hypogonadism (Jockenhorel, Rehrbach, Deggerich, Reinwein, & Reiners, 1996).

Patients with juvenile or adult-onset diabetes mellitus may have low bone mass; however, it is not clear that diabetes is directly related to higher incidence of fragility fractures (Forst et al., 1995). Complications from poorly managed diabetes, including malnutrition, loss of calcium and phosphorus in urine, acidosis, and other metabolic problems may ultimately cause low bone mass (Gregorio, Cristallini, Santeusanio, Filipponi, & Fumelli, 1994;

Munoz-Torres, Jodar, Escobar-Jimenez, Lopez-Ibarra, & Luna, 1996). There may be microvascular defects of osteoblast function. Although there does appear to be increased risk of fracture in type I diabetes, it may be totally unrelated to low bone mass (Katayama, Akatsu, Yamamoto, Kugai, & Nagata, 1996; Seeley, Kelsey, Jergas, & Nevitt, 1996).

Calcium deficiency may be a risk factor for the development of low bone mass, but it may not be the only cause. Certainly, low bone mass may be associated with steatorrhea, biliary cirrhosis, alcoholism, gastrectomy, intestinal bypass, inflammatory bowel disease, gluten sensitive enteropathy, or other chronic gastrointestinal diseases. There may be a combination of both osteomalacia and osteoporosis in these patients.

Other chronic illnesses, including chronic renal disease, rheumatic disease, autoimmune diseases, malignancy, metastatic bone disease, various drugs and toxins, nutritional deficiencies, granulomatous diseases, genetic disorders, immobilization, etc., may mimic primary osteoporosis (Orlic & Raisz, 1999). Vitamin D deficiency is especially common in the elderly and most easily treated with oral supplementation (see next chapter).

Workup for secondary causes should be directed at treatable causes, which may or may not be clinically apparent. It is generally believed that initial screening should include serum and urinary calcium, and serum creatinine. Abnormalities will direct further evaluation (Orlic & Raisz, 1999). For example, with hypercalcemia or hypercalciuria, one should exclude hyperparathyroidism, thyroid disease, multiple myeloma, and granulomatous diseases. With hypocalcemia or hypocalciuria, one should exclude vitamin D deficiency, malabsorption, chronic liver disease, and chronic renal disease. With normal serum and urine calcium, particularly in premenopausal women and in men, one should consider evaluation for hypogonadism. Thyroid function studies, complete blood count, and serum protein electrophoresis are frequently part of evaluation in elderly populations. One should direct evaluation of secondary causes based on findings from the initial history and physical exam, particularly in the face of chronic renal disease.

An approach to the evaluation and management of the postmenopausal and recently menopausal patient has been suggested by this author (see Figures 7.1–7.3).

INSURANCE COVERAGE OF BMD

With the new legislation passed by the Health Care Financing Administration (HCFA) regulations, which went into effect July 1, 1998, we now have

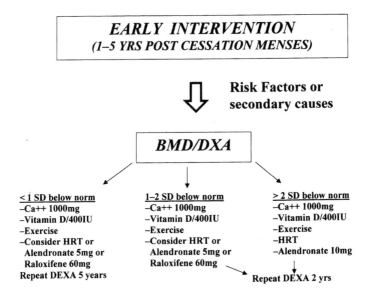

FIGURE 7.2   **Early intervention.**

a uniform coverage for bone mass measurements in the Medicare population, otherwise known as the Bone Mass Measurement Act (BMMA). The law defines "bone mass measurement" as a procedure approved by the Food and Drug Administration (FDA) for the purpose of identifying bone mass, detecting bone loss, and interpreting bone quality in a "qualified individual."

MEDICARE—REIMBURSABLE BMD TECHNIQUES

Measuring Peripheral Skeleton

BONE DENSITOMETRY

- SXA
- pDXA
- RA (radiographic absorptiometry)
- pQCT (peripheral quantitative computer tomography)
- SPA (single photon absorptiometry)

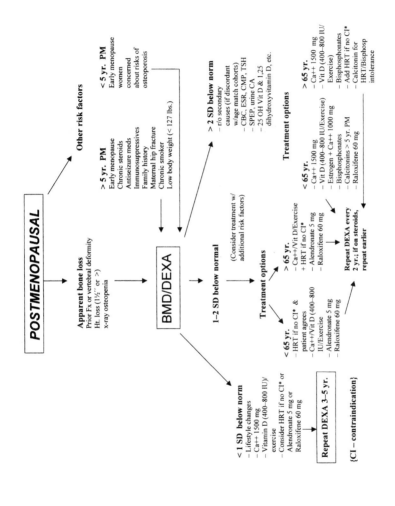

POSTMENOPAUSAL

Apparent bone loss
Prior Fx or vertebral deformity
Ht. loss (1½" or >)
x-ray osteopenia

Other risk factors

>5 yr. PM
Early menopause
Chronic steroids
Antiseizure meds
Immunosuppressives
Family history
Maternal hip fracture
Chronic smoker
Low body weight (<127 lbs.)

<5 yr. PM
Early menopause
women
concerned
about risks of
osteoporosis

BMD/DEXA

1–2 SD below normal
(Consider treatment w/
additional risk factors)

>2 SD below norm
– r/o secondary
  causes (if discordant
  w/age match cohorts)
– CBC, ESR, CMP, TSH
– SPEP, urine CA
– 25 OH Vit D & 1,25
  dihydroxyvitamin D, etc.

<1 SD below norm
– Lifestyle changes
– Ca++ 1500 mg
– Vitamin D (400–800 IU/)
  exercise
– Consider HRT if no CI* or
  Alendronate 5 mg or
  Raloxifene 60 mg

Repeat DEXA 3–5 yr.

{CI – contraindication}

Treatment options

<65 yr.
– HRT if no CI* &
  patient agrees
– Ca++/Vit D (400–800
  IU/Exercise
– Alendronate 5 mg
– Raloxifene 60 mg

>65 yr.
– Ca++/Vit D/Exercise
  + HRT if no CI*
– Alendronate 5 mg
– Raloxifene 60 mg

**Repeat DEXA every
2 yr.; if on steroids,
repeat earlier**

Treatment options

<65 yr.
– Ca++ 1500 mg
– Vit D (400–800 IU/Exercise)
– Estrogen + Ca++ 1000 mg
– Bisphosphonates
– Calcitonins >5 yr. PM
– Raloxifene 60 mg

>65 yr.
– Ca++ 1500 mg
– Vit D (400–800 IU/
  Exercise)
– Bisphosphonates
– Add HRT if no CI*
– Calcitonin for
  HRT/Bisphosp
  intolerance

FIGURE 7.3   Postmenopausal management.

79

BONE SONOGRAPHY

- QUS (quantitative ultrasound)

Measuring Central Skeleton

- DXA (dual energy x-ray absorptiometry)
- QCT (quantitative computer tomography)

Definition of "Qualified Individual"

- An estrogen-deficient woman at clinical risk of osteoporosis as determined by a physician or qualified nonphysician practitioner based on her medical history and other findings
- A person with vertebral abnormalities as demonstrated by x-ray to be indicative of osteoporosis, osteopenia, or vertebral fracture
- A person receiving or expecting to receive long-term glucocorticoid (steroid) therapy (equivalent to greater than or equal to 7.5 mg of prednisone per day for more than 3 months)
- A person with primary hyperparathyroidism
- A person being monitored to assess the response to, or efficacy of, an FDA-approved osteoporosis drug therapy

MEDICARE STANDARDS FOR FREQUENCY OF BMD COVERAGE

General Rule

- Follow-up coverage for BMD measurements will be limited to one test every 2 years (greater than or equal to 23 months since last BMD test). Exceptions include:

  - ◆ More frequent BMD monitoring for persons on long-term (more than 3 months) glucocorticoid (steroid) therapy
  - ◆ More frequent BMD monitoring for other medically necessary conditions (determined by a physician)

◆ A confirmatory baseline BMD measurement will be allowed if BMD monitoring in the future will be performed with a different method than the one used initially

Note that this coverage is applicable immediately and may vary with the local Medicare carrier. For the non-Medicare individual, particularly in the case of the postmenopausal female under 65 years of age, the National Osteoporosis Foundation guidelines recommend BMD testing with at least one additional risk factor for osteoporosis other than menopause should be followed.

In conclusion, currently 28 million Americans are at risk for fracture due to low bone mass, and in excess of 1.5 million fractures occur annually at a cost of approximately $14 billion. With the predictions of exponential cost increases in the future for this "epidemic" disease, it is imperative that health care providers take a proactive approach toward early intervention after early diagnosis. It is expected that guidelines for the evaluation and treatment of osteoporosis, particularly for causes other than postmenopausal, will continue to evolve, making possible the ability to eradicate this disease state entirely.

REFERENCES

Adachi, J. D., Bensen, W. G., Brown, J., Hanley, D., Hodsman, A., Josse, R., Kendler, D. L., Lentle, B., Olszynski, W., Ste-Marie, L. G., Tenenhouse, A., & Chines, A. A. (1997). Intermittent etidronate therapy to prevent corticosteroid-induced osteoporosis. *New England Journal of Medicine, 337,* 382–387.

Adinoff, A. D., & Hollister, J. R. (1983). Steroid-induced fractures and bone loss in patients with asthma. *New England Journal of Medicine, 309,* 265–268.

Arlot, M. E., Sornay-Rendu, E., Garnero, P., Vey-Marty, B., & Delmas, P. D. (1997). Apparent pre- and postmenopausal bone loss evaluated by DXA at different skeletal sites in women: The OFELY cohort. *Journal of Bone Mineral Research, 2,* 683–690.

Bilezikian, J. P., Morishima, A., Bell, J., & Grumbach, M. M. (1998). Increase bone mass as a result of estrogen therapy in a man with aromatase deficiency. *New England Journal of Medicine, 339,* 599–602.

Black, D. M., Cummings, S. R., Genant, H. K., Nevitt, M. C., Palermo, L., & Browner, W. (1992). Axial and appendicular bone density predict fractures in older women. *Journal of Bone Mineral Research, 7,* 633–638.

Blake, G. M., Patel, R., & Fogelman, I. (1998). Peripheral or axial bone density measurements? *Journal of Clinical Densitometry, 1,* 55–65.

Cameron, J. R., & Sorenson, J. (1963). Measurements of bone mineral in vivo: An improved method. *Science, 142,* 230–232.

Canalis, E. (1996). Mechanisms of glucocorticoid action in bone: Implications to glucocorticoid-induced osteoporosis. *Journal of Clinical Endocrinology and Metabolism, 81,* 3441–3447.

Cann, C. E. (1987). Quantitative computed tomography for bone mineral analysis: Technical considerations. In H. K. Genant (Ed.), *Osteoporosis update 1987* (pp. 131–144). San Francisco, CA: University of California Printing Services.

Compston, J. E., Cooper, C., & Kanis, J. A. (1995). Bone densitometry in clinical practice. *British Medical Journal, 310,* 1507–1510.

Consensus Development Conference (1993). *American Journal of Medicine, 94.*

Cummings, S. R., Black, D. M., Nevitt, M. C., Browner, W., Cauley, J., Ensrud, K., Genant, H. K., Palermo, L., Scott, J., & Vogt, T. M. (1993). Bone density at various sites for prediction of hip fractures: The study of osteoporotic fractures research group. *Lancet, 341,* 72–75.

Cummings, S. R., Black, D. M., Nevitt, M. C., Browner, W. S., Cauley, J. A., Genant, H. K., Mascioli, S. R., Scott, J. C., Seeley, D. G., & Steiger, P. (1990). Appendicular bone density and age predict hip fracture in women. *Journal of American Medical Association, 263,* 665–668.

Cummings, S. R., Black, D. M., & Rubin, S. M. (1989). Lifetime risks of hip, Colles', or vertebral fracture and coronary heart disease among white postmenopausal women. *Archives of Internal Medicine, 149,* 2445–2448.

Cummings, S. R., Black, D. M., & Vogt, T. M. (1996). Changes in BMD substantially underestimate the anti-fracture effects of alendronate and other antiresorptive drugs. *Journal of Bone Mineral Research, 11*(Suppl. 1), S102.

Drinka, P. J., DeSmet, A. A., Bauwens, S. F., & Rogot, A. (1992). The effect of overlying calcification on lumbar bone densitometry. *Calcified Tissue International, 50,* 507–510.

Dunn, W. L., Wahner, H. W., & Riggs, B. L. (1980). Measurement of bone mineral content in human vertebrae and hip by dual photon absorptiometry. *Radiology, 136,* 485–487.

Evans, J., & Tavakoli, M. (1990). Ultrasonic attenuation and velocity in bone. *Physics in Medicine and Biology, 35,* 1387–1396.

Forst, T., Pfutzner, A., Kann, P., Schehler, B., Lobmann, R., Schafer, H., Andreas, J., Bockisch, A., & Beyer, J. (1995). Peripheral osteopenia in adult patients with insulin-dependent diabetes mellitus. *Diabetic Medicine, 12,* 874–879.

Frye, M. A., Melton, L. J. III, Bryant, S. C., Fitzpatrick, L. A., Wahner, H. W., Schwartz, R. S., & Riggs, B. L. (1992). Osteoporosis and calcification of the aorta. *Journal of Bone and Mineral Research, 19,* 185–194.

Gardsell, P., Johnell, O., & Nilsson, B. E. (1991). The predictive value of bone loss for fragility fractures in women: A longitudinal study over 15 years. *Calcified Tissue International, 49,* 90–94.

Genant, H. K., Block, J. E., Steiger, P., & Gluer, C. (1987). Quantitative computed tomography in the assessment of osteoporosis. In H. K. Genant (Ed.), *Osteoporosis update 1987* (pp. 49–72). San Francisco, CA: University of California Printing Services.

Genant, H. K., Cann, C. E., Ettinger, B., & Gordan, G. S. (1982). Quantitative computed tomography of vertebral spongiosa: A sensitive method for detecting early bone loss after oophorectomy. *Annals of Internal Medicine, 97,* 699–705.

Gluer, C., Vahlensieck, M., Faulkner, K., Engelke, K., Black, D., & Genant, H. (1992). Site-matched calcameal measurements of broad-band ultrasound attenuation and single x-ray absortiometry: Do they measure different skeletal properties? *Journal of Bone Mineral Research, 7,* 1071–1079.

Greenspan, S. L., Maitland-Ramsey, L., & Myers, E. (1996). Classification of osteoporosis in the elderly is dependent on site-specific analysis. *Calcified Tissue International, 58,* 409–414.

Gregorio, F., Cristallini, S., Santeusanio, F., Filipponi, P., & Fumelli, P. (1994). Osteopenia associated with non-insulin dependent diabetes mellitus: What are the causes? *Diabetes Research and Clinical Practice, 23,* 43–54.

Hans, D., Dargent-Molina, P., Schott, A. M., Sebert, J. L., Cormier, C., Kotzki, P. O., Delmas, P. D., Pouilles, J. M., Breart, G., & Meunier, P. J. (1996). Ultrasonographic heel measurements to predict hip fracture in elderly women: The EPIDOS prospective study. *Lancet, 348,* 511–514.

Hawker, G. A. (1996). The epidemiology of osteoporosis. *The Journal of Rheumatology, 23*(Suppl. 45), 2–5.

Hui, S. L., Slemenda, C. W., & Johnston, C. C. Jr. (1988). Age and bone mass as predictors of fracture in a prospective study. *Journal of Clinical Investigation, 81,* 1804–1809.

Hui, S. L., Slemenda, C. W., & Johnston, C. C. Jr. (1989). Baseline measurement of bone mass predicts fracture in white women. *Annals of Internal Medicine, 111,* 355–361.

Jockenhorel, F., Rehrbach, S., Deggerich, S., Reinwein, D., & Reiners, C. (1996). Differential presentation of cortical and trabecular peripheral bone mineral density in acromegaly. *European Journal of Medical Research, 1,* 377–382.

Kalender, W. A. (1992). Effective dose values in bone mineral measurements by photon absortiometry and computed tomography. *Osteoporosis International, 2,* 82–87.

Kanis, J. A. (1994). Osteoporosis and its consequences. In R. Marcus (Ed.), *Osteoporosis* (pp. 1–6). Boston, MA: Blackwell Scientific.

Kanis, J. A. (1994). Osteoporosis and its consequences. In R. Marcus (Ed.), *Osteoporosis* (p. 8). Boston, MA: Blackwell Scientific.

Kanis, J. A. (1994). Osteoporosis and its consequences. In R. Marcus (Ed.), *Osteoporosis* (pp. 1–20). Boston, MA: Blackwell Scientific.

Katayama, Y., Akatsu, T., Yamamoto, M., Kugai, N., & Nagata, N. (1996). Role of nonenzymatic glycosylation of type 1 collagen in diabetic osteopenia. *Journal of Bone Mineral Research, 11,* 931–937.

Kelly, T. L., Slovik, D. M., Schoenfeld, D. A., & Neer, R. M. (1988). Quantitative digital radiography versus dual photon absorptiometry of the lumbar spine. *Journal of Clinical Endocrinology and Metabolism, 67,* 839–844.

Krane, S. M., & Holick, M. (1994). Metabolic bone disease. *Harrison's Principles of Internal Medicine, 358,* 2172–2177.

Langton, C., Evans, G., Hodgskinson, R., & Riggs, C. (1990). Ultrasonic, elastic and structural properties of cancellous bone. In Current Research in Osteoporosis and Bone Mineral Measurements. *British Institute of Radiology* 10–11.

Leb, G., Warnkross, H., & Obermayer-Pietsch, B. (1994). Thyroid hormone excess and osteoporosis. *Acta Medica Austriaca, 21,* 5–67.

Lees, B., & Stevenson, J. C. (1992). An evaluation of DXA and comparison with dual-photon absorptiometry. *Osteoporosis International, 2,* 146–152.

Lems, W. F., Van Veen, G. J., Gerrits, M. I., Jacobs, W. G., Houben, H., Van Rijn, H., & Bijlsma, J. (1988). Effect of low dose prednisone (with calcium and calcitriol supplementation) on calcium and bone metabolism in healthy volunteers. *British Journal of Rheumatology, 37,* 27–33.

Mack, P. B., O'Brien, A. T., Smith, J. M., & Bauman, A. W. (1939). A method for estimating degree of mineralization of bones from tracings of roentgenograms. *Science, 89,* 467.

Mazess, R. B., Barden, H., Ettinger, M., & Schulz, E. (1988). Bone densitometry of the radius, spine, and proximal femur in osteoporosis. *Journal of Bone Mineral Research, 3,* 13–18.

Melton, L. J. III, Atkinson, E. J., O'Fallon, W. M., Wahner, H. W., & Riggs, B. L. (1993). Long-term fracture prediction by bone mineral assessed at different skeletal sites. *Journal of Bone Mineral Research, 8,* 1227–1233.

Miller, P. D., & McClung, M. (1996). Prediction of fracture risk I: Bone density. *American Journal of Medical Science, 312,* 257–259.

Miller, P. D., Bonnick, S. L, Johnston, C. C., Kleerekoper, M., Lindsay, R. L., Sherwood, L. M., & Siris, E. S. (1998). The challenges of peripheral bone density: Which patients need additional central density skeletal measurements? *American Journal of Medical Science, 1,* 211–217.

Munoz-Torres, M., Jodar, E., Escobar-Jimenez, F., Lopez-Ibarra, P. J., & Luna, J. D. (1996). Bone mineral density measured by dual x-ray absorptiometry in Spanish patients with insulin-dependent diabetes mellitus. *Calcified Tissue International, 58,* 316–319.

National Osteoporosis Foundation. (1998). *Physician's guide to prevention and treatment of osteoporosis.* Belle Mead, NJ: Excerpta Medica.

Nelson, D. A., Molley, R., & Kleerekoper, M. (1998). Prevalence of osteoporosis in women referred for bone density testing. *Journal of Clinical Densitometry, 1,* 5–11.

Nguyen, T. V., Sambrook, P. N., & Eisman, J. A. (1997). Sources of variability in bone mineral density measurements: Implications for study design and analysis of bone loss. *Journal of Bone Mineral Research, 12,* 124–135.

Orlic, Z. C., & Raisz, L. G. (1999). Causes of secondary osteoporosis. *Journal of Clinical Densitometry, 2,* 79–92.

Povilles, J. M., Tremollieres, R., & Ribot, C. (1993). Spine and femur densitometry at menopause: Are both sites necessary in the assessment of the risk of osteoporosis? *Calcified Tissue International, 52,* 344–347.

Povilles, J. M., Tremollieres, F., Todorovsky, N., & Ribot, C. (1991). Precision and sensitivity of DXA in spinal osteoporosis. *Journal of Bone Mineral Research, 6,* 997–1002.

Ray, N. F., Chan, J. K., Thamer, M., & Melton, L. J. III. (1997). Medical expenditures for the treatment of osteoporotic fracture in the United States in 1995: Report from the National Osteoporosis Foundation. *Journal of Bone Mineral Research, 12,* 24–35.

Reid, I. R. (1997). Glucocorticoid osteoporosis: Mechanisms and management. *European Journal of Endocrinology, 137,* 209–217.

Reid, I. R. (1997). Preventing glucocorticoid-induced osteoporosis. *New England Journal of Medicine, 337,* 420–421.

Riggs, B. L., & Melton, L. J. III. (1995). The worldwide problem of osteoporosis: Insights afforded by epidemiology. *Bone, 17*(Suppl. 5), 5055–5115.

Ross, P. D. (July, 1996). Osteoporosis, frequency, consequences, and risk factors. *Archives of Internal Medicine, 156,* 1399–1411.

Ross, P. D., Davis, J. W., Epstein, R. S., & Wasnich, R. D. (1991). Pre-existing fractures and bone mass predict vertebrae fracture incidence in women. *Annals of Internal Medicine, 114,* 919–923.

Ross, P., Huang, C., Davis, J., Imose, K., Yates, J., Vogel, J., & Wasnich, R. (1995). Predicting vertebral deformity using bone densitometry at various skeletal sites and culcaneal ultrasound. *Bone, 16,* 325–332.

Saag, K. G., Emkey, R., Schnitzer, T. J., Brow, J. P., Hawkins, F., Goemaere, S., Thamsborg, G., Liberman, U. A., Delmas, P. D., Malice, M. P., Czachur, M., & Daifotis, A. G. (1998). Alendronate for the prevention and treatment of glucorticoid-induced osteoporosis. *New England Journal of Medicine, 339,* 292–299.

Seeley, D. G., Kelsey, J., Jergas, M., & Nevitt, M. C. (1996). Predictors of ankle and foot fractures in older women: The study of osteoporotic fractures research group. *Journal of Bone Mineral Research, 11,* 1347–1355.

Slemenda, C. W., Hui, S. L., Longcope, C. (1990). Predictors of bone mass in perimenopausal women. *Annals of Internal Medicine, 112,* 96–101.

Tavakoli, M., & Evans, J. (1991). Dependence of the velocity and attenuation of ultrasound in bone on the mineral content. *Physics in Medicine and Biology, 36,* 1529–1537.

U.S. Congress (1994). *Hip fracture outcomes* (OTA-BP-H-120).

Vanderscheueren, D., & Bouillon, R. (1995). Androgens and bone. *Calcified Tissue International, 56,* 341–346.

Wahner, H. W., Dunn, W. L., Mazess, R. B., Towsley, M., Lindsay, R., Markhard, L., & Dempster, D. (1983). Dual photon Gd-152 absorptiometry of bone. *Radiology, 156,* 203–206.

Wasnich, R. (1993). Bone mass measurement: Prediction of risk. *American Journal of Medicine, 95*(Suppl. 5A), 6S–10S.

Wasnich, R. D., Ross, P. D., Heilbrun, L. K., & Vogel, J. M. (1985). Prediction of postmenopausal fracture risk with use of bone mineral measurements. *American Journal of Obstetrics and Gynecology, 153,* 745–751.

Yates, A. J., Ross, P. D., Lydick, E., & Epstein, R. (1995). Radiographic absorptiometry in the diagnosis of osteoporosis. *American Journal of Medicine, 98*(Suppl. 2A), 415–475.

8

Therapeutic Strategies for Prevention and Treatment

M. Susan Burke

It's never too early nor too late to institute nonpharmacologic strategies.

—M. S. Burke

In postmenopausal osteoporosis, there are two main groups of women to target for intervention. One is the recently postmenopausal woman who has not yet lost a significant amount of bone mass. She has osteopenia and will benefit from nonpharmacologic and pharmacologic therapy to help her *maintain* as high a bone mass as possible and *prevent* bone loss. The other woman is more easily identified. She has already fractured, lost height, or been found to have visible osteopenia or a compression fracture on x-ray. Her bones are fragile, and she is much more likely to have another fracture. This osteoporotic patient requires agents that *build* bone mass, *treat* her weakened bones, and *reduce* her future fracture rate. The purpose of this chapter is to review the therapies presently available to achieve these prevention and treatment goals.

NONPHARMACOLOGIC PREVENTION AND TREATMENT

Nonpharmacologic therapy consists of calcium, vitamin D, and exercise. *All* patients of *all* ages can benefit from this—it is never too early nor too late to institute these measures. If begun early enough and continued throughout life, they help increase peak bone mass and reduce the rate of bone loss with aging. When administered to osteoporotic patients, their effect to slow bone loss tends to decrease fracture rates compared to those not on treatment, but they generally do not build bone mass. Therefore, it is important to reiterate that *once osteopenia or osteoporosis develops, pharmacologic therapy will be needed to build bone mass and reduce fracture risk.*

Calcium

As described in the section on bone remodeling, the skeleton not only requires calcium for proper mineralization but also serves as a reservoir, a calcium bank of sorts, to maintain proper serum calcium levels. Adequate nutritional intake of calcium throughout life reduces the need to "withdraw" bone calcium to meet this need. This equates to better bone health, as patients with lifelong high calcium intake have been demonstrated to have fewer hip fractures than those with low intake (Matkovic et al., 1979).

The recommended requirements of calcium vary depending on age, sex, and estrogen status and are listed in Table 8.1. Because estrogen enhances the gastrointestinal absorption of calcium, postmenopausal women not on

TABLE 8.1 Recommendation for Daily Calcium Intake (in Milligrams of Elemental Calcium)

Population	RDA	NIH/NOF	IOM
Children			
1–10 years		800–1,200 mg	
9–18 years			1,300 mg
Men and women			
25–64 years	800 mg	1,000 mg	
Pregnant/lactating	1,200 mg		
Postmenopausal with HRT		1,000 mg	1,200 mg
Over age 65–70		1,500 mg	1,200 mg

hormone replacement therapy need a higher calcium intake. Milk and other dairy products are the major sources of calcium. Others include calcium-fortified orange juice, collard and turnip greens, tofu, oysters, and broccoli. It is unusual for adequate calcium intake to be attained by diet alone. Many patients try to avoid the extra calories and cholesterol associated with dairy products. The recent increase in calcium fortified cereals, breads, etc., can help some patients achieve the recommended daily requirement, but often a patient would still benefit from a calcium or calcium plus vitamin D supplement. Examples of various calcium products available are shown in Table 8.2.

CLINICAL ISSUES

Note that the daily calcium requirement refers to milligrams of *elemental* calcium. Calcium carbonate is often the cheapest and has the best percentage of elemental calcium (40%). Some calcium formulations are better tolerated by a particular patient than others, so try different ones, if necessary. Have

TABLE 8.2 Selected Calcium/Calcium +D Supplements

Supplement	Total (mg)	Elemental (mg)	Vitamin D (IU)
	Calcium carbonate (40% elemental calcium)		
Tums	500	200	
Tums Ex	750	300	
Tums 500	1,250	500	
Oscal	1,250	500	
Oscal-D	1,250	500	125 IU
Caltrate	1,500	600	
Caltrate-D	1,500	600	200 IU
Viactiv Soft Chews[a]	1,250	500	100 IU
Calburst	1,250	500	200 IU
	Calcium citrate (21% elemental calcium)		
Citracal Liquitabs	2,376	500	
Citracal 1,500	1,500	315	
Citracal 1,500 + D	1,500	315	200 IU
	Calcium phosphate (39% elemental calcium)		
Posture	1,500	600	
Posture-D	1,500	600	125 IU

[a]Also contains 40 mg vitamin K.

the patient take calcium carbonate with meals, if possible. The extra acid enhances its absorption. Calcium citrate is recommended if the patient is achlorhydric.

Divide the dose of calcium throughout the day, since only so much is absorbed at one time. However, it is probably more important that a patient take it all at once than to forget some doses. Evening doses may help reduce the nocturnal increase in bone resorption.

Not all calcium supplements are created equal. Although most brand name supplements are tested and proven to be absorbed clinically, some inexpensive generic brands have not. To check the tablet's absorption, have the patient put it into one-fourth cup vinegar (roughly equivalent to stomach acid). It should fully dissolve in one-half hour; if it does not, the patient can see this and realize that it will not be effective.

VITAMIN D

Background

Vitamin D_3 is produced in the skin on exposure of 7-deoxycholesterol (provitamin D_3) to ultraviolet B sunlight. It enters the circulation and is hydroxylated in the liver to $25(OH)D_3$. Under the influence of serum calcium levels and PTH, $25(OH)D_3$ is again hydroxylated to $1,25(OD_2)D_3$, the active form of vitamin D. Its action is to maintain proper calcium levels by enhancing intestinal absorption of calcium and stimulating osteoclasts to resorb bone.

Aging decreases the amount of provitamin D_3 in the skin. For example, a person over age 70 makes less than 30% of the vitamin D_3 manufactured by the skin of a young adult (Holick, Matsuoka, & Wortsman, 1989). In addition, factors such as season of the year, time of daily sun exposure, and latitude can significantly influence vitamin D_3 levels. Patients living in more northern areas may go many months without meaningful skin production of vitamin D_3, and this can lead to a decrease in bone mineral density during the winter that partially or completely rebounds in the summer (Rosen et al., 1994).

Vitamin D deficiency is a fairly common finding in older patients, contributing to the secondary hyperparathyroidism seen in some older women. Up to 60% of patients with hip fractures may have an element of vitamin D deficiency (Lips et al., 1982). Although studies of supplementation with vitamin D alone do not demonstrate fracture reduction (Lips, Graafmans, Ooms, Bezemer, &

Bouter, 1996), supplementation of vitamin D plus calcium reduces the rate of bone loss, may increase bone mass (Chapuy et al., 1992), and decrease the incidence of hip and other nonvertebral fractures (Dawson-Hughes, Harris, Krall, & Dallal, 1997).

Vitamin D occurs naturally in fatty fish and fish oils and is a fortified ingredient in milk. However, to assure adequate amounts, it is recommended that all older patients receive vitamin D supplementation. Recent studies suggest that the RDA for vitamin D should be 600-800 IU, especially for older adults (Holick, 1994). Doses above 1,000 IU are not recommended and can be toxic.

CLINICAL ISSUES

The use of sunscreen (as low as factor 8 protection) may eliminate skin production of vitamin D (Holick, 1994).

It is best to administer vitamin D as part of a multivitamin, or as a calcium plus vitamin D supplement (see Table 8.2). Patients should not rely exclusively on milk for vitamin D supplementation. One study revealed that less than 50% of milk samples from various dairies contained the amount specified on the label (Holick, Shao, Liu, & Chen, 1992).

EXERCISE

Part of the reason that bone grows and remodels is in response to the mechanical stresses that it handles. Increased load increases bone mass; decreased load decreases bone mass. Lack of stress, as in complete immobilization, results in considerable bone loss—up to 40% of the individual's starting bone mass in one year (Marcus, 1996, p. 254).

The type of exercise influences the amount of bone mass increase. Although low load, repetitive weight-bearing exercises (walking, jogging, climbing stairs, dancing, racket sports) stimulate bone growth, much greater growth is achieved with higher load, low repetition exercises (weight lifting, leg press, jumping). Specific exercises for specific skeletal sites, especially the upper extremity, are recommended so that all areas may benefit from stimulation. Tennis players, for example, have been shown to have a higher bone mineral density in their racket-holding forearm than their ball-tossing forearm (Huddleston, Rockwell, Kulund, & Harrison, 1980).

All patients, no matter what age, can profit from some type of exercise. The benefit may be an increase in bone mass, better cardiovascular health, or improved gait and balance. In fact, the enhanced muscle strength achieved with even mild exercise will reduce the risk for falling and decrease the chance that a fracture will occur.

OTHER LIFESTYLE FACTORS

For multiple health reasons, patients should be encouraged to stop smoking. Women smokers reach menopause with about 10% less bone mass than nonsmokers (Hopper & Seeman, 1994). Smoking accelerates the degradation of estrogen and also results in some decrease in bone formation through an unknown mechanism. Thirty years of smoking roughly doubles a woman's fracture risk.

Alcohol abuse also inhibits bone formation, possibly due to a direct toxic effect on osteoblasts. The decrease in bone mass and increase in fracture rate is more common in men than in women because of alcohol's additional adverse effect on testicular function. Moderate alcohol intake is not usually associated with lower bone density except perhaps in lower weight patients.

Many elements and minerals such as magnesium, manganese, copper, zinc, vitamin C, and vitamin K are required for proper bone synthesis and mineralization, although their requisite amounts have not been determined. Vitamin K, for example, is necessary for the γ carboxylation of bone matrix proteins such as osteocalcin. It may also act to decrease urinary calcium excretion. It is reasonable for all patients to maintain proper diet, and to use a complete supplement (such as Centrum) if they are at high risk.

PHARMACOLOGIC PREVENTION AND TREATMENT

Pharmacologic *prevention* therapy is indicated for the recently postmenopausal woman at high risk for osteoporosis (thin build, maternal history of fracture, failure to achieve peak bone mass, etc., as outlined in chapter 6). Therapy may be started in these patients without necessarily obtaining a bone mineral density (BMD) test, particularly if the patient agrees to take hormone replacement therapy. If not performed at the start of therapy, it should be obtained some time during the next two to four years to assess the therapy's effectiveness. Pharmacologic prevention therapy is also indicated for a postmenopausal woman of any age who is found to have osteopenia (T-score between −1 and −2 to −2.5 SD below the mean). This patient, if left untreated, is at high risk for fractures in her remaining lifetime. The goals of prevention therapy in all these patients are to *maintain* bone mass, *prevent* further bone loss, and *reduce* fracture risk. Agents approved for osteoporosis prevention are hormone replacement therapy (estrogen), alendronate 5 mg (a bisphosphonate), and raloxifene (a selective estrogen receptor modulator, or SERM).

Pharmacologic *treatment* therapy is indicated for patients found to have osteoporosis either because they have already fractured or because they are found to have a T-score ≤ -2 or -2.5 S.D. below the mean by central BMD measurement. Here, the goals of treatment are to increase bone mass, prevent further bone loss, and reduce the risk of a first fracture or additional fractures. A T-score of -2 or the presence of a single vertebral fracture increases vertebral fracture risk five-fold and also increases the risk of hip fracture. Because the personal and economic cost of a hip or vertebral fracture can be so devastating, medication should be administered as early as possible to reduce this risk. Therapies indicated for osteoporosis treatment are hormone replacement therapy, alendronate 10 mg, raloxifene, and calcitonin. Each therapeutic agent will now be addressed.

HORMONE REPLACEMENT THERAPY

Mechanism of Action

Prior to menopause, estrogen exerts an inhibitory effect on osteoclasts and a stimulatory effect on osteoblasts. During this time, bone mass is generally constant or decreases somewhat after age 30. The loss of estrogen at menopause, however, can result in significant bone loss. In the five years after menopause, a woman may lose up to one third of the bone mass she is destined to lose in her remaining lifetime. Administration of estrogen restores its beneficial influence on bone remodeling, with the net effect being an increase in bone mass.

Indications: Prevention and Treatment

PREVENTION

As a prevention therapy for the postmenopausal or osteopenic patient, estrogen replacement reduces the amount of bone loss and generally leads to an increase in bone mass. In most studies, estrogen increases lumbar BMD

TABLE 8.3 Estrogens Approved for Prevention and/or Treatment

Agent	Conjugated estrogens (CE) — Alone: Premarin[a]	With medroxyprogesterone acetate (MPA): Prempro	With medroxyprogesterone acetate (MPA): Premphase	Estropipate: Ogen[a]	Esterified estrogens: Estratab, Manest[a]	Estrace[a]	17B Estradiol: Climara[a]	17B Estradiol: Estraderm[a]
Indication	Prevention and treatment	Prevention and treatment	Prevention	Prevention	Prevention	Prevention	Prevention	Prevention
Route of administration	Oral	Oral	Oral	Oral	Oral	Oral	Transdermal	Transdermal
Regimen	Daily	Daily 0.625 mg Conj. Estrogen + 2.5 mg MPA daily for full 28-day cycle	Daily 0.625 mg Conj. Estrogen X 28 days + 5.0 mg MPA on days 15–28 of each cycle	Daily	Daily	Daily	Once weekly	Twice weekly
Available strengths	0.3 mg 0.625 mg 0.9 mg 1.25 mg 2.5 mg			0.625 mg 1.25 mg 2.5 mg	0.3 mg 0.625 mg 1.25 mg 2.5 mg	1 mg 2 mg	0.05 mg 0.075 mg 0.1 mg	0.05 mg 0.1 mg

[a]Must be combined with medrosyprogesterone acetate or norethindrone acetate either cyclically or continuously in patients with an intact uterus.

approximately 4–5%, and hip BMD approximately 3% over 2 years. As the prototypical prevention agent, it should be offered to every woman at the time of menopause if there are no contraindications. In a woman with an intact uterus, it must be given with progesterone either cyclically or continuously. Estrogen therapy should be started as close as possible to the onset of menopause to help maintain as high a bone mass as possible. However, even women in their eighth decade may reduce their bone loss with estrogen replacement (Lindsay, Hart, & Clark, 1984). Similar results were seen in the Rancho Bernardo study (Schneider, Barrett-Connor, & Morton, 1997), which evaluated the effects of timing and duration of estrogen therapy on BMD. This cross-sectional study demonstrated that the highest bone densities were achieved when estrogen was started at the time of menopause and continued indefinitely. However, estrogen begun and continued after age 60 offered nearly as much beneficial effect as long-time usage. Past users exhibited little or no remaining bone preservation benefit because of the rapid decrease in bone density with discontinuation of estrogen replacement (Schneider et al., 1997). Therefore, *for optimal bone sparing benefit, estrogen therapy should commence at the time of menopause and be continued indefinitely.*

TREATMENT

Estrogen is a recommended treatment for osteoporosis in the patient who has already fractured, as well as for the patient found to be osteoporotic by x-ray or BMD testing. It is believed that estrogen reduces fractures of the hip, wrist, and spine. The actual reduction, however, is not known, and current estimates of fracture reduction are based primarily on retrospective studies. Dose, timing, and duration of estrogen use with respect to menopause are all confounding variables. Generally, estrogen reduces fractures 35%–60%, with greater benefits seen in those who began estrogen at the time of menopause, those who are presently on estrogen, or those on it for a longer duration (Cauley, Salamone, & Lucas, 1996, p. 561). One small prospective study involving 75 postmenopausal patients with at least one vertebral fracture reported a 61% decrease in new fractures with the use of estrogen for one year compared to placebo (Lufkin et al., 1992).

Although estrogen is considered the gold standard for osteoporosis prevention, not all patients experience an increase in bone mass. Because of this, the National Osteoporosis Foundation recommends BMD testing for all women on long-term hormone replacement to assure that the patient has responded to this treatment (*Physician's Guide to Prevention and Treatment of Osteoporosis,*

1998, p. 13). Recent studies utilizing hormone replacement and alendronate together demonstrate additive bone benefits (Greenspan et al., 1998). This combination should be considered in patients who have not responded adequately to estrogen therapy or in those found to have very low bone mass.

CLINICAL ISSUES

Controversy still exists over the detrimental effects of long-term estrogen administration (> 10 years) on the incidence of breast cancer. Concerns on the part of the patient as well as the physician tend to hinder its long-term use. Although one study showed that there may be an increased incidence of breast cancer in women who use hormone replacement, both the size of the tumor as well as the mortality from these lesions were actually reduced in the hormone users (Sellers et al., 1997). The decision to initiate estrogen therapy in women with established cardiovascular disease is also being questioned. The Heart and Estrogen/Progesterone Replacement Study (HERS) prospectively evaluated this combination compared to placebo in women with established coronary disease. After 4 years, no reduction in cardiovascular events was demonstrated; in fact, the estrogen/progestin users had an increased number of these events during the first year of the trial. Although not a primary endpoint, the incidence of fractures was not decreased in the estrogen group; it should be noted, however, that the women in this study were less osteoporotic and it is more difficult to demonstrate fracture reduction in such patients (Hulley et al., 1998). The NIH-sponsored Woman's Health Initiative is a large prospective study designed to answer many questions related to estrogen replacement, but results will not be available for several years.

Dosing

There are many formulations of estrogen available (see Table 8.4). Most studies demonstrating increases in bone mass and reduction in fractures used 0.625 mg of conjugated estrogen or its equivalent. It is easier to give this dose to the recently postmenopausal patient whose system is used to having this hormone. The older woman should be started on a lower dose to reduce side effects, but there is less information concerning low doses and fracture protection. A recent study (Recker, Davies, Dowd, & Haeney, 1999) demonstrated a bone-sparing effect of continuous administration of 0.3 mg conjugated

**TABLE 8.4 Approved Agents for Prevention
and/or Treatment of Osteoporosis**

Agent	Indication	Dose	BMD increase	Fracture reduction
Estrogen (Premarin, Estrace, etc.)	Prevention	0.3–0.625 mg CE or its equivalent	4%–5% spine and 3% hip in 2 years	
	Treatment	0.625–1.25 mg CE or its equivalent		~35–60% spine- and hip-fracture reduction (pooled analysis)[a]
Alendronate (Fosamax)	Prevention	5 mg	3.5% spine and 1.9% in hip in 2 years[b]	
	Treatment	10 g	8.8% spine and 6%–7.8% hip in 3 years[c]	55% reduction in clinically apparent spine fractures, 51% reduction in hip fractures[d], 48% reduction in wrist fractures[d]
Calcitonin (Miacalcin, Calcimar)	Treatment (for women > 5 years after menopause)	200 I.U. intranasally, 100 S.C. or i.m.	2%–3% spine in 2 years	18%–34% reduction in vertebral fractures[e]
Raloxifene (Evista)	Prevention and treatment	60 mg	2.4% spine and 2.4% hip in 2 years[f]	30% reduction in vertebral fractures[g]

Note: These are not head to head studies.
[a]From Cauley et al. (1996).
[b]From Hosking et al. (1998).
[c]From Liberman et al. (1995).
[d]From Black et al. (1996).
[e]From Maricic et al. (1998).
[f]From Delmas et al. (1997).
[g]From Ettinger et al. (1999).

estrogen and 2.5 mg medroxyprogesterone in elderly women comparable to other studies using higher doses. The effect of this regimen on fracture rate is not known. Therefore, it is still suggested that the dose be slowly titrated to the equivalent of at least 0.625 mg of conjugated estrogens if possible. A repeat bone mineral density test in two years is recommended, and adequate calcium and vitamin D should also be administered.

If the patient has not had a hysterectomy, progesterone must also be administered to reduce the risk of endometrial cancer due to estrogen induced proliferation of the uterine lining. This can be done cyclically, with estrogen 0.625 mg administered on days 1–25, and medroxyprogesterone 10 mg given on days 12–25. Days 26–30/31 have no hormones administered. This results in some monthly spotting and is not tolerated by many patients. A more popular regimen is continuous estrogen/progesterone therapy of 0.625 mg/2.5 mg daily. There is initial sporadic spotting for 2 to 3 months until the endothelial lining atrophies. If it persists, an increase in the progesterone to 5 mg daily should help. Rarely, 10 mg/day of progesterone may be necessary.

ALL patients must have a baseline mammogram, Pap, and pelvic exam. *Once amenorrhea is achieved with continuous therapy, any new vaginal bleeding deserves evaluation.*

Side Effects

Most patients are familiar with the side effects of estrogen use, which reduce long-term compliance. These include breast tenderness, vaginal bleeding, fluid retention, exacerbation of migraine headaches, and weight gain. Increasing the dose slowly may lessen some of these unpleasant side effects. Despite this, long-term compliance with hormone replacement is poor, with up to 80% of patients not continuing treatment past three years. Fortunately, if it is declined or not tolerated, other pharmacologic therapies are now available.

Contraindications to Estrogen Replacement

There are several absolute contraindications to estrogen use: presence or history of breast cancer, two first-degree relatives with breast or ovarian cancer, endometrial cancer within the last three years, history of current thrombophlebitis, or prior thrombophlebitis related to pregnancy or oral contraceptive use, and unexplained vaginal bleeding. Relative contraindications include chronic hepatocellular dysfunction, history of gall bladder disease, and elevated triglycerides.

ALENDRONATE

Mechanism of Action

Because HRT is not always tolerated or indicated in all women, investigators looked to other agents to prevent and treat postmenopausal bone loss. Alendronate is one of several bisphosphonates that has been studied for this purpose. It is attracted to and binds strongly with the calcium phosphate found in bone mineral. When an osteoclast becomes stimulated to resorb bone, it engulfs the alendronate, which interferes with the cholesterol pathway within the osteoclast. Consequently, osteoclast function is impaired and the cell undergoes apoptosis (cell death) (Fleisch, 1997). Bone formation by osteoblasts is unaffected, and the net result is an increase in bone density.

Indications: Prevention and Treatment

PREVENTION

Alendronate at the 5 mg dose is indicated to prevent osteoporosis. In the Early Postmenopausal Interventional Cohort Study (Hosking et al., 1998), the use of alendronate was compared to HRT and to placebo to see if comparable bone-sparing effects could be achieved with this nonhormonal agent. Alendronate was found to increase BMD 3.5% in the lumbar spine and 1.9% in the hip, and was better tolerated than HRT (Hosking et al., 1998). At the 5 mg dose, alendronate is an attractive alternative for postmenopausal women who cannot or will not take estrogen. It is indicated for the same patient groups described in HRT prevention therapy: the postmenopausal patient at risk, and the osteopenic patient.

TREATMENT

At present, alendronate at the 10 mg dose has documented the most evidence for reducing the fractures and subsequent disability of osteoporosis compared to the other available agents. In the Fracture Intervention Trial (FIT) (Black et al., 1996), women with at least one vertebral fracture were randomized to receive placebo or alendronate for three years (5 mg the first two years; 10 mg the third year, when this dose was found to be more beneficial). The study was terminated early because of the compelling evidence for fracture reduction. Clinically apparent vertebral fractures were reduced 55%, hip fractures by 51%, and wrist fractures by 48% (Black et al., 1996). Overall, the group receiving alendronate had a 20% incidence reduction in hospitalizations and a 28% reduction in emergency room visits. A comparable reduction in fractures of the spine and hip is seen in other studies (Liberman et al., 1995). The Fosamax International Trial (FOSIT) (Pols et al., 1999) evaluated the effect of 10 mg alendronate daily on fracture rate in women with a lumbar spine T-score of 2 or more standard deviations (SD) below the young adult mean. A 47% reduction in nonvertebral fractures was demonstrated after one year, and this effect could be noticed beginning at three months of therapy (Pols et al., 1999). Another arm of FIT assessed the effects of alendronate (5 mg for the first two years, 10 mg for the next two years) in women with osteopenia or osteoporosis who had not yet fractured. Vertebral and hip fractures were reduced in the subset of women whose T-score was < −2. In women whose score was > −2, no reduction in fractures was seen (Cummings et al., 1998), suggesting that it may take longer to demonstrate fracture benefit in patients who do not have severe bone loss.

Dosing

The prevention dose is 5 mg daily, the treatment dose is 10 mg daily. Alendronate should be continued indefinitely. Although discontinuation of alendronate does not result in the rapid bone loss seen with HRT discontinuation, a gradual decline does occur, so some maintenance therapy should be utilized. The dosing may be modified once optimal bone mass is restored. One could then consider reducing the 10 mg dose to the 5 mg prevention dose daily, or perhaps to 10 mg every other day. A once weekly dose of 70 mg or a twice weekly dose of 35 mg is presently being evaluated as an alternative dosing regimen but has not yet been approved. Adequate calcium and vitamin D should also be administered.

Alendronate must be taken first thing in the morning on an empty stomach with eight ounces of plain water. Because bisphosphonates are poorly absorbed, the patient must wait at least one-half hour before eating anything, including coffee or juice. Certain medications like thyroxine may be administered with the alendronate. Reflux of the acid-bisphosphonate mixture may induce esophageal irritation, and anything that worsens reflux, such as lying down, must be avoided.

CLINICAL ISSUES

Unfortunately, there are many perceptions about the use of alendronate—its adverse effects, taking it in the morning without food, etc.—that inhibit its use and keep some patients from benefiting from it. Practitioners have found the following methods helpful in enhancing compliance:

1. Consider starting all patients on the 5 mg dose for 2 to 3 weeks. Advise the patient that this will allow her "stomach lining to get used to it," before increasing to the 10 mg dose.
2. Have the patient keep the drug on the nightstand and take it as soon as possible after rising.
3. Ask the patient what her morning routine is before offering this medicine. She may very well do other things for at least a half hour before she begins eating. One could even say how nicely alendronate's dosing would fit into her routine. If she eats soon after rising, suggest some things she could do during this time.
4. Have the patient take a sip of water first to moisten the esophagus if she has trouble swallowing pills. Room temperature water may induce less esophageal spasm. The patient could keep the water on the nightstand for use the next morning.

If the patient experiences gastrointestinal symptoms, consider these options before switching medications:

1. If calcium supplements were recently added, make sure those are not the culprit. Calcium carbonate in particular may induce bloating, gas, and abdominal discomfort. This seems particularly true with Oscal. Caltrate is generally better tolerated.
2. If it does not seem to be due to calcium, discontinue the alendronate and have the patient take a prescription strength H_2 blocker such as famotidine or ranitidine, or a proton pump inhibitor such as omeprazole every evening for a few weeks. Restart alendronate at the 5 mg dose daily or every other day while continuing the acid-suppressing agent. Animal studies have shown that if the pH of the gastric contents is higher, less esophageal irritation develops (Peter, Handt, & Smith, 1998).

3. If the above measures fail, consider giving the total weekly dose as a single dose or split into a twice weekly dose. Although not yet an approved regimen, the benefits to the patient may exceed those from the use of other agents.

Adverse Effects

In the various clinical trials of alendronate, the incidence of adverse effects, including esophageal, gastric, and other abdominal events were comparable to placebo. A study of alendronate-induced esophagitis found that most of the patients who developed this problem had not complied with the dosing regimen, either by not using enough water (6–8 oz.), not staying upright for one half hour, or not discontinuing the medication at the onset of severe symptoms (de Groen et al., 1996). Patients must be instructed to discontinue the medication if they develop trouble swallowing, retrosternal pain, or new or worsening heartburn. If the patient develops minor discomfort while on alendronate, temporarily discontinuing the drug and advising them about some of the techniques listed in clinical issues section may be helpful.

Contraindications

The use of alendronate is contraindicated in patients with abnormalities of the esophagus such as stricture, achalasia, dysmotility, and Barrett's esophagus. Because of the importance of remaining upright for one half hour to prevent significant reflux, alendronate is not indicated for anyone who is unable to do this. Bedbound patients and patients with active upper gastrointestinal diseases such as recent or recurrent ulcers or UGI bleeding should not be given this drug. In addition, alendronate is not recommended for patients with a creatinine clearance < 35 ml/min, and patients with hypocalcemia.

Patients with gastroesophageal reflux disease (GERD) may take alendronate if their symptoms are controlled with antireflux therapy. Also, patients with a prior history of ulcers that are not presently active may also be given alendronate with appropriate follow-up.

CALCITONIN

Mechanism of Action

In 1962, calcitonin was recognized as a hormone secreted by the C-cells of the thyroid gland that can decrease plasma calcium concentration. The therapeutic action of calcitonin is not completely understood. It primarily inhibits osteoclast activity by altering cytoplasmic motility with resultant slowing of bone resorption (Chambers & Dunn, 1983). Calcitonin receptors are also present on osteoblasts, so this hormone may exert some action on bone formation (Wallach, Farley, Baylink, & Brenner-Gati, 1993). Additionally, calcitonin increases renal calcium excretion. The therapeutic formulation used is salmon calcitonin; it is 50–100 times more potent than human calcitonin.

Indication: Treatment

Calcitonin is indicated for treatment of postmenopausal osteoporosis in women who are five or more years past menopause who cannot or will not take hormone replacement. This agent has been available for treatment of osteoporosis for over 15 years in the injectable form, and over 4 years in the intranasal form. Well designed, long-term clinical studies with appropriate numbers of patients have not yet been completed (Civitelli, 1996, p. 1240). In a time when the outcome of a therapeutic intervention should drive its use, the efficacy of this agent in fracture reduction has yet to be adequately demonstrated. Because of these considerations, calcitonin is presently viewed as a third-line agent if hormone replacement and alendronate cannot be used (*Physician's Guide to Prevention and Treatment of Osteoporosis*, 1998, p. 21).

Calcitonin increases bone mass in the vertebral spine by approximately 2%–3% in one year, with attenuation of further response thereafter. It is not known whether this is due to antibody formation or to a limitation of the number of remodeling spaces that calcitonin can influence. Most studies show no significant increase in cortical bone of the wrist or hip. What investigations have been carried out have not been powered to assess fracture reduction, and the results have been varying and inconsistent. All must be interpreted carefully because of small study size and design problems, high dropout rates, and questions concerning patient randomization (Civitelli, 1996, p. 1240). The Proof of Recurrent Osteoporotic Fractures Trial (PROOF) (Maricic et al., 1998), a recently completed five-year trial designed to assess the efficacy of calcitonin to reduce vertebral fractures, randomized 1,255 postmenopausal women with established osteoporosis to receive either placebo, 100 IU, 200 IU (the FDA approved dose), or 400 IU of intranasal calcitonin. Three hundred seventy-eight patients completed the study. The vertebral fracture reduction reported was between 18%–36% but was not dose-dependent. No effect on hip fractures was noted (Maricic et al., 1998).

However, a European retrospective study of over 5,000 patients found an approximately 30% decrease in the relative risk of hip fracture in women who had received calcitonin (Kanis et al., 1992).

Dosing

Intranasally, the dose is 200 IU daily in alternating nostrils. When used parenterally (intramuscularly or subcutaneously), a small test dose should be administered first to minimize the risk of severe allergy or anaphylaxis. Although the optimal dose to prevent loss of vertebral bone mass has not been determined, a dose of 100 IU s.c. or i.m. every other day is generally used. Adequate calcium and vitamin D should also be administered.

CLINICAL ISSUES

Calcitonin has been found to be beneficial in reducing the acute pain associated with vertebral fractures in some studies (Lyritis, Tsakalakos, Magiasis, Karachalios, & Yiatzides, 1991). Others have found this action to be overestimated (Haas, Liebrich, & Schaffner, 1990) or have noted the intranasal administration to be associated with a more rapid onset of action of pain relief than the i.m. form or placebo at two weeks, but comparable to i.m. or placebo by four weeks. The mechanism of action has not been well defined, but is probably mediated through central opioid receptors rather than a direct effect on bone.

Adverse Effects

Calcitonin is generally well-tolerated. Side effects of the intranasal form include rhinitis in about 12%, epistaxis in 3.5%, and sinusitis in 2.3% of patients. Periodic examination of the nose is recommended. With the parenteral form, patients may experience occasional anorexia, nausea, vomiting, metallic taste, flushing, and diarrhea.

Contraindications

Calcitonin is contraindicated in patients who have a hypersensitivity to it.

RALOXIFENE

Mechanism of Action

Raloxifene belongs to a relatively new class of agents known as the selective estrogen receptor modulators or SERMs. These drugs bind to the estrogen receptors throughout the body. Their design allows them to act like estrogen (agonist) on certain receptors while having an anti-estrogen, or blocking effect (antagonist), on others. Raloxifene exerts estrogen agonistic effects on bone and low-density and total cholesterol. Like estrogen, it inhibits osteoclast activity, thus reducing bone resorption and allowing formation to continue. It does not relieve the symptoms of menopause, so it may not be well-tolerated in patients with hot flashes.

Raloxifene, formerly keoxifene, was originally investigated as a treatment for breast cancer. Although it is less potent than tamoxifen in blocking breast cancer cell growth (Gottardis & Jordan, 1987), it may have a preventive effect on breast cancer development, and this is being evaluated in clinical trials (Cummings et al., 1998).

Just as estrogen interacts with receptors throughout the body, a SERM like raloxifene does as well. Although raloxifene decreases total and LDL cholesterol, it does not increase HDL or triglycerides as estrogen does. There is beginning evidence that estrogens delay the onset of Alzheimer's Disease. It is not known what influence raloxifene may have on this condition. Raloxifene's effect on ovary, colon, vascular lining, and other areas with estrogen receptors also needs to be evaluated in long-term human studies in order to understand the full effects of this agent. In rats, for example, ovarian tumors were increased in the raloxifene-treated animals (Evista (Raloxifene) tablets' product monograph [package insert].

Indications: Prevention and Treatment

PREVENTION

Raloxifene is indicated for prevention of osteoporosis in recently postmenopausal women or postmenopausal women of any age with osteopenia. In a 24-month study, 60 mg of raloxifene was found to increase both lumbar spine and total hip BMD by 2.4% compared to placebo, and 1%–1.5% compared to baseline (Delmas et al., 1997), a more modest effect than that seen with estrogen or alendronate. A 10% decrease in LDL cholesterol was noted, and no increase in endometrial thickness by transvaginal ultrasonography was detected.

TREATMENT

Based on the vertebral fracture reductions seen in the MORE study (Multiple Outcomes of Raloxifene Evaluation), raloxifene at the 60 mg dose received approval for treatment of osteoporosis. In this study 7,705 women with post-menopausal osteoporosis with or without baseline vertebral fractures were randomized to placebo, 60 mg (the FDA-approved dose), or 120 mg of raloxifene. On the 60 mg dose, women experienced a 30% incidence reduction in vertebral fracture; no reduction in nonspine fractures was demonstrated (Ettinger et al., 1999). An additive effect on the increase in BMD and decrease in markers of bone turnover can be seen with the combination of raloxifene and alendronate at one year (Johnell, Scheele, Lu, & Lakshinanan, 1999).

DOSING

The recommended dose is 60 mg daily without regard to meals. Concurrent use of cholestyramine is not recommended since it markedly reduces raloxifene's bioavailability. Patients on coumadin should have their prothrombin time (PT) monitored—the PT may decrease up to 10%. Since raloxifene is highly protein bound, caution should be taken when coadministering other protein bound drugs such as naproxen, indomethacin, ibuprofen, diazepam, clofibrate, or diazoxide.

Clinical Issues

The antagonistic effects that raloxifene exerts on breast and uterine tissue make this agent an alternative for patients with a personal or strong family history of breast cancer who desire some of estrogen's benefits. It can also be considered for others not willing to take estrogen or not able to tolerate alen-dronate.

ADVERSE EVENTS

The most common side effects of this drug are hot flashes and leg cramps. The hot flashes are generally of mild or moderate severity and can be attributed to its anti-estrogen effect on this symptom. The etiology of the leg cramps is not known, but does not seem to be related to mineral imbalance, vascular, or muscular damage. The incidence of thrombotic events (deep venous thrombosis, pulmonary embolism, or retinal vein thrombosis) is approximately twice that seen with estrogen, the greatest risk occurring within the first four months of treatment. Raloxifene should be discontinued at least 72 hours prior to surgery and during prolonged periods of immobilization (Evista package insert, Eli Lilly, 1997).

CONTRAINDICATIONS

Raloxifene is contraindicated in premenopausal women, and may cause fetal harm if administered during pregnancy. It should not be administered to women with a history of venous thrombotic events, those currently on estrogen, or women with a known hypersensitivity to it. Raloxifene is metabolized and excreted primarily by the liver, and its safety in patients with significant liver disease has not been evaluated.

DRUGS IN DEVELOPMENT

Advances in identification and diagnosis of osteoporosis has spurred interest in developing agents to prevent and treat this disease. There are several agents undergoing investigation.

Other Bisphosphonates

Risedronate is an aminobisphosphonate in the same class as alendronate and works in a similar fashion to prevent osteoclast action and reduce bone resorption. It has recently been approved for prevention and treatment of osteoporosis in Sweden. It is expected to receive approval for this use in the United States in the first quarter of 2000. In an early menopausal (prevention) population, 5 mg of risedronate daily for two years was shown to increase bone mass in the lumbar spine by 1.4% and the femoral neck by 1% compared to baseline, and by 5%–6% in both sites compared to placebo (Mortensen, Charles, Bekker, Digennaro, & Johnston, 1998). In postmenopausal women with one or more vertebral fractures, 5 mg of risedronate daily for three years decreased the rate of new vertebral fractures by 41% and nonspine fractures by 39% (Harris et al., 1999; Watts et al., 1999).

Etidronate has been available for years as a treatment for Paget's disease and has been used for treatment of osteoporosis despite the fact that it is not approved for this indication in the United States. In controlled trials, etidronate increases bone mass in the spine and hip and reduces vertebral fractures, especially in patients with very low bone mass (Harris et al., 1993). As a nonnitrogen-containing bisphosphonate, it is not specific for osteoclasts, and therefore inhibits both osteoclast and osteoblast activity. Because of this, etidronate has a much narrower therapeutic-to-toxic ratio than the newer bisphosphonates and must be dosed cyclically to prevent inhibition of mineralization. A 400 mg dose is given daily 2 hours before breakfast for 2 weeks, followed by 10–13 weeks of 500 mg calcium daily. When used in this manner, it is safe and well tolerated.

Pamidronate, ibandronate, clodronate, and tiludronate are other bisphosphonates under investigation for postmenopausal osteoporosis.

Fluoride

Unlike the other agents available for prevention and treatment which inhibit bone resorption, fluoride is the only drug available that stimulates bone formation. Despite the fact that fluoride induces large increases in BMD, earlier studies of fluoride demonstrated no effect or even an increase in fracture rate (Riggs et al., 1990). These studies generally used large doses of fluoride, which can result in osteomalacia. More recent small studies using intermittent doses of a slow-release sodium fluoride showed that it decreased new vertebral fractures but not recurrent ones (Pak et al., 1994). Continuous low dose fluoride at 20 mg daily with calcium may decrease vertebral fractures compared with calcium alone (Reginster et al., 1998). Fluoride treatment can be associated with gastric irritation and may induce stress fractures. Because of the availability of other efficacious agents, fluoride treatment is not presently recommended.

Parathyroid Hormone

Human PTH is being evaluated as a therapeutic modality in osteoporosis. Although known to increase bone turnover, PTH also can stimulate new bone formation. In preliminary studies, PTH induces dramatic increases in spinal BMD when used in combination with estrogen and may decrease fracture rates compared to estrogen (Lindsay et al., 1997).

Ipraflavone

Ipraflavone is a synthetic derivative of isoflavones. These are compounds synthesized by plants and found to have estrogenic properties. Ipraflavone appears to inhibit osteoclastic activity and reduce osteoclast precursors, and preliminary studies demonstrate increases in bone mass (Brandi, 1996). It is under investigation in several countries, including the U.S.

Finally, vitamin D analogues, other SERMS like droloxifene, and strontium salts are among the agents in development to treat osteoporosis.

THERAPEUTIC STRATEGIES FOR SPECIAL SITUATIONS

Male Osteoporosis

Men are not immune to the progressive bone loss that occurs with aging. According to the National Health and Nutrition Examination Survey (NHANES III 1988–91) osteoporosis is present in 6% and osteopenia in 47% of males over age 50. As the life expectancy in the United States increases, one can anticipate this disease to increase in both sexes. The male:female ratio of vertebral fractures has been calculated to be 1:2 (Cooper, Atkinson, O'Fallon, & Melton, 1992) and the hip fracture ratio approaches 1:3 (Cooper, Champion, & Melton, 1992).

Age is the most important risk for male osteoporosis, with a peak 10–15 years later than postmenopausal osteoporosis. Except for menopause, risk factors for male osteoporosis are similar to those in women. Excessive alcohol use may be a more important risk. Since other etiologies for decreased bone mass may be present in up to 30% of cases, some secondary workup is warranted. It is similar to that outlined in chapter 7 and should include a testosterone level. Although men do not experience the dramatic decline in sex hormones that women have at menopause, there is some age-related decline in testosterone levels, a 75-year-old male having only two-thirds the level of a 25-year-old (Vermuelen, Rubens, & Verdonck, 1972). Men who experience hip or vertebral fractures are more likely to have decreased testosterone levels than those who have not fractured.

Just as for women, adequate calcium, vitamin D, and exercise should be encouraged. If the testosterone level is found to be low, intramuscular or transdermal testosterone will increase bone mass, this treatment will not help those with normal testosterone levels. It is reasonable to expect that the nonhormonal therapies available for postmenopausal osteoporosis should work similarly in males, and a recently completed study of alendronate for male osteoporosis demonstrated significant BMD increases, similar to those seen in women (Weber & Dregner, 1999). An indication for its use in this population is expected shortly. Calcitonin may be considered third line if the above treatments are not tolerated.

Steroid-Induced Osteoporosis

Although prednisone is a vital therapy for many inflammatory conditions, it results in a two to five times higher risk of fracture, and can affect any age group. Glucocorticoids exert this adverse influence in a variety of ways. Their main action is to inhibit osteoblast activity by reducing their function and life span. They also stimulate PTH and subsequent osteoclast activity. Calcium's absorption from the GI tract and reabsorption from the renal tubule is also reduced. Finally, the decrease in corticotropin and gonadotropin during steroid administration results in decreased sex hormone production in men and women, further compounding the imbalance between bone resorption and formation.

Dramatic decreases in BMD may result from even low doses of prednisone –7.5 mg or its equivalent, and the decrease can begin almost immediately. The effect is most severe in the first 6–12 months of treatment, when up to 15% of bone mass may be lost. Therefore, *prevention of bone resorption should be initiated when the steroid prescription is first written.* The American College of Rheumatology has issued guidelines on preventing steroid-induced osteoporosis (American College of Rheumatology Task Force on Osteoporosis Guidelines, 1996).

Recommendations for the prevention and treatment of glucocorticaid-induced osteoporosis.

1. Use the lowest dose of steroids possible. Alternate day dosing does not prevent bone loss.
2. Use inhaled or topical steroids if possible.
3. Make sure the patient consumes 1,500 mg calcium daily through diet or supplementation. This should be instituted at the start of steroid therapy.
4. Prescribe vitamin D at 800 IU daily.

5. Prescribe HRT for women if not contraindicated.
6. Prescribe bisphosphonates or calcitonin if: HRT is contraindicated, refused, or if osteoporosis develops despite the measures just described.

Since the publication of these guidelines, alendronate has received the indication to treat steroid-induced osteoporosis and should be considered for all patients in whom long-term steroid administration is contemplated. In a 48-week trial of men and women on steroid therapy, both 5 and 10 mg of alendronate were shown to increase bone mass in the spine and hip (Saag, Emkey, Schnitzer, et al., 1998). The 10 mg dose was more effective in women who were not on hormone replacement therapy. In a small extension study of this trial, new vertebral fractures were found to be significantly reduced in those randomized to alendronate therapy (Saag, Emkey, Cividino, et al., 1998).

Administration of testosterone to men whose testosterone levels are affected by steroid therapy may increase BMD in the lumbar spine by 5% in 12 months (Reid, Wattie, Evans, & Stapleton, 1996). Etidronate increases bone mass in steroid users, but to a lesser extent than alendronate, and does not appear to be as protective at the hip (Roux et al., 1998). Calcitonin may also prevent steroid-induced bone loss (Luengo et al., 1990). As with postmenopausal osteoporosis, however, the data with calcitonin is not always consistent; and some studies show no significant effect on BMD or fracture rate in steroid-dependent patients (Healey et al., 1996).

REFERENCES

American College of Rheumatology Task Force on Osteoporosis. (1996). Recommendations for the prevention and treatment of glucocorticoid-induced osteoporosis. *Arthritis and Rheumatism, 39,* 1791–1801.

Black, D. M., Cummings, S. R., Karpf, D. B., Cauley, J. A., Thompson, D. E., Nevitt, M. C., Bauer, D. C., Genant, H. K., Haskell, W. L., Marcus, R., Ott, S. M., Torner, J. C., Quandt, S. A., Reiss, T. F., & Ensrud, K. E. (1996). Randomised trial of effect of alendronate on risk of fracture in women with existing vertebral fractures. *Lancet, 348,* 1535–1541.

Brandi, M. L. (1996). Ipraflavone: In vitro and in vivo effects on bone metabolism. In R. Marcus, D. Feldman, & J. Kelsey (Eds.), *Osteoporosis* (pp. 1335–1344). New York: Academic Press.

Cauley, J. A., Salamone, L. M., & Lucas, F. L. (1996). Postmenopausal endogenous and exogenous hormones, degree of obesity, thiazide, diuretics, and risk of osteoporosis. In R. Marcus, D. Feldman, & J. Kelsey (Eds.), *Osteoporosis* (p. 561). New York: Academic Press.

Chambers, T. J., & Dunn, C. J. (1983). Pharmacological control of osteoclastic motility. *Calcified Tissue International, 35,* 566–579.

Chapuy, M. C., Arlot, M. E., Duboeuf, F., Brun, J., Crouzet, B., Arnaud, S., Delmas, P. D., & Meunier, P. J. (1992). Vitamin D3 and calcium to prevent hip fractures in elderly women. *New England Journal of Medicine, 327,* 1637–1642.

Civitelli, R. (1996). Calcitonin. In R. Marcus, D. Feldman, & J. Kelsey (Eds.), *Osteoporosis* (p. 1240). New York: Academic Press.

Cooper, C., Atkinson, E. J., O'Fallon, W. M., & Melton, L. J., III. (1992). Incidence of clinically diagnosed vertebral fractures: A population-based study in Rochester, Minnesota 1985–1989. *Journal of Bone and Mineral Research, 7,* 221–227.

Cooper, C., Champion, G., & Melton, L. J., III. (1992). Hip fractures in the elderly: A world-wide project. *Osteoporosis International, 2,* 285–289.

Cummings, S. R., Norton, L., Eckert, S., Grady, D., Cauley, J., Knickerbocker, R., Black, D. M., Nickelsen, T., Glusman, J., & Krueger, K. (1998). Raloxifene reduces the risk of breast cancer and may decrease the risk of endometrial cancer in postmenopausal women: Two-year findings from the multiple outcomes of raloxifene evaluation (MORE) trial. *Proceedings of the American Society of Clinical Oncology Meeting, 3.*

Dawson-Hughes, B., Harris, S. S., Krall, E. A., & Dallal, G. E. (1997). Effect of calcium and vitamin D supplementation on bone density in men and women 65 years of age or older. *New England Journal of Medicine, 337,* 670–676.

de Groen, P. C., Lubbe, D. F., Hirsch, L. J., Daifotis, A., Stephenson, W., Freedholm, D., Pryor-Tillotson, S., Seleznick, M. J., Pinkas, H., & Wang, K. K. (1996). Esophagitis associated with the use of alendronate. *New England Journal of Medicine, 335,* 1016–1021.

Delmas, P. D., Bjarnason, N. H., Mitlak, B. H., Ravoux, A. C., Shah, A. S., Huster, W. J., Draper, M., & Christiansen, C. (1997). Effects of raloxifene on bone mineral density, serum cholesterol concentrations, and uterine endometrium in postmenopausal women. *New England Journal of Medicine, 337,* 1641–1647.

Ettinger, B., Black, D., Mitlak, B., Knickerbocker, R., Nickelsen, T., Genant, H., Christiansen, C., Delmas, P., Zanchetta, J., Stakkestad, J., Gluer, C., Krueger, K., Cohen, F., Eckert, S., Ensrud, K., Avioli, L., Lips, P., & Cummings, S. (1999). Reduction of vertebral fracture risk in postmenopausal osteoporosis treated with raloxifene: Results from a three-year randomized, clinical trial. *Journal of the American Medical Association, 282,* 637–645.

EU CPMP. (1998, August). *European Public Assessment Report,* CPMP/1070/98.

Fleisch, H. (1997). *Bisphosphonates in bone disease: From the laboratory to the patient* (3rd ed.). New York: Parthenon Publishing.

Gottardis, M. M., & Jordan, V. C. (1987). Antitumor actions of keoxifene and tamoxifen in the N-nitrosomethylurea-induced rat mammary carcinoma model. *Cancer Research, 47,* 4020–4024.

Greenspan, S., Bankhurst, A., Bell, N., Bolognese, M., Bone, H., Davidson, M., Downs, R., Emkey, R., McKeever, C., Miller, S., Mulloy, A., Weiss, S., Heyden, N., Lombardi, A., & Suryawanshi, S. (1998). Effects of alendronate and estrogen alone or in combination on bone mass and turnover in postmenopausal osteoporosis. *ASBMR-IBMS Second Joint Meeting*, S174. (Abstract No. 1108).

Haas, H. G., Liebrich, B. M., & Schaffner, W. (1990). Calcitonin and osteoporosis: A critical review of the literature. *Klinische Wochenschrift, 68*, 359–371.

Harris, S., Watts, N., Genant, H., McKeever, C., Hangartner, T., Keller, M., Chestnut, C., Brown, J., Eriksen, E., Hoseyni, M., Axelrod, D., & Miller, P. (1999). Effects of risedronate treatment on vertebral and nonvertebral fractures in women with postmenopausal osteoporosis: A randomized, controlled trial. *Journal of the American Medical Association, 282*, 1334–1352.

Harris, S. T., Watts, N. B., Jackson, R. D., Genant, H. K., Wasnich, R. D., Ross, P., Miller, P. D., Licata, A. A., & Chesnut, C. H. III. (1993). Four-year study of intermittent cyclic etidronate treatment of postmenopausal osteoporosis: Three years of blinded therapy followed by one year of open therapy. *American Journal of Medicine, 95*, 557–567.

Healey, J. H., Paget, S. A., Williams-Russo, P., Szatrowski, T. P., Schneider, R., Spiera, H., Mitnick, H., Ales, K., & Schwartzberg, P. (1996). A randomized controlled trial of salmon calcitonin to prevent bone loss in corticosteroid-treated temporal arteritis and polymyalgia rheumatica. *Calcified Tissue International, 58*, 73–80.

Holick, M. F. (1994). Vitamin D: New horizons for the 21st century. *American Journal of Clinical Nutrition, 60*, 619–630.

Holick, M. F., Matsuoka, L. Y., & Wortsman, J. (1989). Age, vitamin D, and solar radiation. *Lanet, 4*, 1104–1105.

Holick, M. F., Shao, Q., Liu, W. W., & Chen, C. C. (1992). The vitamin D content of fortified milk and infant formula. *New England Journal of Medicine, 326*, 1178–1181.

Hopper, J. L., & Seeman, E. (1994). The bone density of twins discordant for tobacco use. *New England Journal of Medicine, 330*, 387–392.

Hosking, D., Chilvers, C. E., Christiansen, C., Ravn, P., Wasnich, R., Ross, P., McClung, M., Balske, A., Thompson, D., Daley, M., & Yates, A. J. (1998). Prevention of bone loss with alendronate in postmenopausal women under 60 years of age. *New England Journal of Medicine, 338*, 485–492.

Huddleston, A. L., Rockwell, D., Kulund, D. N., & Harrison, R. B. (1980). Bone mass in lifetime tennis athletes. *Journal of the American Medical Association, 244*, 1107–1109.

Hulley, S., Grady, D., Bush, T., Furberg, C., Herrington, D., Riggs, B., & Vallinghoff, E. (1998). Randomized trial of estrogen plus progesterone for secondary prevention of coronary heart disease in postmenopausal women [Heart and Estrogen/Progesterone Replacement Study (HERS) Research Group]. *Journal of the American Medical Association, 280,* 605–613.

Johnell, O., Scheele, W., Lu, Y., Lakshinanan, M. (1999). Effects of raloxifene, alendronate and raloxifene, and alendronate on bone mineral density and biochemical markers of bone turnover in postmenopausal women with osteoporosis. *ASBMR 21st Annual Meeting.* (Abstract No. 1100).

Kanis, J. A., Johnell, O., Gullberg, B., Allander, E., Dilsen, G., Gennari, C., Lopes Vaz, A. A., Lyritis, G. P., Mazzuoli, G., Miravet, L., Passeri, M., Cano, R. P., Rapado, A., & Ribot, C. (1992). Evidence for efficacy of drugs affecting bone metabolism in preventing hip fracture. *British Medical Journal, 305,* 1124–1128.

Liberman, U. A., Weiss, S. R., Broll, J., Minne, H. W., Quan, H., Bell, N. H., Rodriguez-Portales, J., Downs, R. W., Jr., Dequeker, J., & Favus, M. (1995). Effect of oral alendronate on bone mineral density and the incidence of fractures in postmenopausal osteoporosis. *New England Journal of Medicine, 333,* 1437–1443.

Lindsay, R., Hart, D. M., & Clark, D. M. (1984). The minimum effective dose of estrogen for the prevention and treatment of postmenopausal bone loss. *Obstetrics and Gynecology, 63,* 759–763.

Lindsay, R., Nieves, J., Formica, C., Henneman, E., Woelfert, L., Shen, V., Dempster, D., & Cosman, F. (1997). Randomised controlled study of effect of parathyroid hormone on vertebral-bone mass and fracture incidence among postmenopausal women on estrogen with osteoporosis. *Lancet, 350,* 550–555.

Lips, P., Graafmans, W. C., Ooms, M. E., Bezemer, P. D., & Bouter, L. M. (1996). Vitamin D supplementation and fracture incidence in elderly persons: A randomized, placebo-controlled clinical trial. *Annals of Internal Medicine, 124,* 400–406.

Lips, P., Netelenbos, J. C., Jongen, M. J., van Ginkel, F. C., Althuis, A. L., van Schaik, C. L., van der Vijgh, W. J., Vermeiden, J. P., & van der Meer, C. (1982). Histomorphometric profile and vitamin D status in patients with femoral neck fracture. *Metabolic Bone Disease and Related Research, 4,* 85–93.

Luengo, M., Picado, C., Del Rio, L., Guanabens, N., Montserrat, J. M., & Setoain, J. (1990). Treatment of steroid-induced osteopenia with calcitonin in corticosteroid-dependent asthma. *American Review of Respiratory Disease, 142,* 104–107.

Lufkin, E. G., Wahner, H. W., O'Fallon, W. M., Hodgson, S. F., Kotowicz, M. A., Lane, A. W., Judd, H. L., Caplan, R. H., & Riggs, B. L. (1992). Treatment of postmenopausal osteoporosis with transdermal estrogen. *Annals of Internal Medicine, 117,* 1–9.

Lyritis, G. P., Tsakalakos, N., Magiasis, B., Karachalios, T., & Yiatzides, A. (1991). Analgesic effect of salmon calcitonin in osteoporotic vertebral fractures: A double-blind placebo-controlled study. *Calcified Tissue International, 49,* 369–372.

Marcus, R. (1996). Physical activity and regulations of bone mass. In M. J. Favus (Ed.), *Primer on the metabolic bone diseases and disorders of mineral metabolism* (3rd ed., p. 254). Philadelphia: Lippincott-Raven.

Maricic, M. J., Silverman, S. L., Chestnut, C., Baylink, D. J., Altman, R., Genant, H. K., Gimona, A., Andriano, K., & Richardson, P. (1998). Salmon-calcitonin nasal spray prevents vertebral fractures in established osteoporosis: Further interim results of the PROOF study. *Arthritis and Rheumatism, 41*(Suppl. 9), 578.

Matkovic, V., Kostial, K., Simonovic, I., Buzina, R., Brodarec, A., & Nordin, B. E. (1979). Bone status and fracture rates in two regions of Yugoslavia. *American Journal of Clinical Nutrition, 32,* 540–549.

Mortensen, L., Charles, P., Bekker, P. J., Digennaro, J., & Johnston, C. C., Jr. (1998). Risedronate increases bone mass in an early postmenopausal population: Two years of treatment plus one year of follow-up. *Journal of Clinical Endocrinology and Metabolism, 83,* 396–402.

National Osteoporosis Foundation. (1998). *Physician's guide to prevention and treatment of osteoporosis.* Belle Meade, NJ: Excerpta Medica.

Pak, C. Y., Sakhaee, K., Piziak, V., Peterson, R. D., Breslau, N. A., Boyd, P., Poindexter, J. R., Herzog, J., Heard-Sakhaee, A., Haynes, S., Adams-Huet, B., & Reisch, J. (1994). Slow-release sodium fluoride in the management of postmenopausal osteoporosis: A randomized controlled trial. *Annals of Internal Medicine, 120,* 625–632.

Peter, C. P., Handt, L. K., & Smith, S. M. (1998). Esophageal irritation due to alendronate sodium tablets: Possible mechanisms. *Digestive Diseases and Sciences, 43,* 1998–2002.

Pols, H. A. P., Felsenberg, D., Hanley, D. A., Stepan, J., Munoz-Torres, M., Wilkin, T. J., Qin-sheng, G., Galich, A. M., Vandormael, K., Yates, A. J., & Stych, B. (1999). Multinational, placebo-controlled, randomized trial of the effects of alendronate on bone density and fracture risk in postmenopausal women with low bone mass: Results of the FOSIT study. *Osteoporosis International, 9,* 461–468.

Recker, R. R., Davies, K. M., Dowd, R. M., & Heaney, R. P. (1999). The effect of low-dose continuous estrogen and progesterone therapy with calcium and vitamin D on bone in elderly women: A randomized, controlled trial. *Annals of Internal Medicine, 130,* 897–904.

Reginster, J. Y., Meurmans, L., Zegels, B., Rovati, L. C., Minne, H. W., Giacovelli, G., Taquet, A. N., Setnikar, I., Collette, J., & Gosset, C. (1998). The effect of sodium monofluorophosphate plus calcium on vertebral fracture rate in postmenopausal women with moderate osteoporosis: A randomized, controlled trial. *Annals of Internal Medicine, 129,* 1–8.

Reid, K. R., Wattie, D. J., Evans, M. C., & Stapleton, J. P. (1996). Testosterone therapy in glucocorticoid-treated men. *Archives of Internal Medicine, 156,* 1173–1177.

Riggs, B. L., Hodgson, S. F., O'Fallon, W. M., Chao, E. Y., Wahner, H. W., Muhs, J. M., Cedel, S. L., & Melton, L. J. III. (1990). Effect of fluoride treatment on the fracture rate in postmenopausal women with osteoporosis. *New England Journal of Medicine, 322,* 802–809.

Rosen, C. J., Morrison, A., Zhou, H., Storm, D., Huster, S. J., Musgrave, K., Chen, T., Wen-Wei, L., & Holick, M. F. (1994). Elderly women in northern New England exhibit seasonal changes in bone mineral density and calciotropic hormones. *Bone and Mineral, 25,* 83–92.

Roux, C., Oriente, P., Laan, R., Hughes, R. A., Ittner, J., Goemaere, S., Di Munno, O., Pouilles, J. M., Horlait, S., & Cortet, B. (1998). Randomized trial of effect of cyclical etidronate in the prevention of corticosteroid-induced bone loss. *Journal of Clinical Endocrinology and Metabolism, 83,* 1128–1133.

Saag, K., Emkey, R., Cividino, A., Brown, J., Goemaere, S., Dumortier, T., Daifotis, A. G., & Czachur, M. (1998). Effects of alendronate for two years on BMD and fractures in patients receiving glucocorticoids. *ASBMR-IBMS Second Joint Meeting,* S182. (Abstract No. 1141).

Saag K. G., Emkey, R., Schnitzer, T. J., Brown, J. P., Hawkins, F., Goemaere, S., Thamsborg, G., Liberman, U. A., Delmas, P. D., Malice, M. P., Czachur, M., & Daifotis, A. G. (1998). Alendronate for the prevention and treatment of glucocorticoid-induced osteoporosis: Glucocorticoid-induced osteoporosis intervention study group. *New England Journal of Medicine, 339,* 292–299.

Schneider, D. L., Barrett-Connor, E. L., & Morton, D. (1997). Timing of postmenopausal estrogen for optimal bone mineral density: The Rancho Bernardo study. *Journal of the American Medical Association, 227,* 543–547.

Sellers, T. A., Mink, P. J., Cerhan, J. R., Zheng, W., Anderson, K. E., Kushi, L. H., & Folsom, A. R. (1997). The role of hormone replacement therapy in the risk for breast cancer and total mortality in women with a family history of breast cancer. *Annals of Internal Medicine, 127,* 973–980.

Vermuelen, A., Rubens, R., & Verdonck, L. (1972). Testosterone secretion and metabolism in late senescence. *Journal of Clinical Endocrinology and Metabolism, 34,* 730–735.

Wallach, S., Farley, J. R., Baylink, D. J., & Brenner-Gati, L. (1993). Effects of calcitonin on bone quality and osteoblastic function. *Calcified Tissue International, 52,* 335–339.

Watts, N., Hangartner, T., Chesnut, C., Genant, H., Miller, P., Eriksen, E., Chines, A., Axelrod, D., & McKeever, C., for the North American Risedronate Osteoporosis Study Group. (1999, May). *Risedronate treatment prevents vertebral and nonvertebral fractures in women with postmenopausal osteoporosis.* Paper presented at the 26th European Symposium on Calcified Tissues (Abstract No. O–24, 524). Maastricht: The Netherlands.

Weber, T., & Dregner, K. (1999). Alendronate increases bone mineral density in male idropathic osteoporosis. *ASBMR 21st Annual Meeting.* (Abstract No. F345).

9

Osteoporosis and Fall Prevention

Roberta Newton

Approximately 30% of adults over 65 years of age and 40% of adults over age 75 years experience at least one fall annually.

—Tinetti, Speechley, & Ginter

Falls are a major cause of injury-related death in individuals over the age of 65 years and are a leading cause of death in older adults over the age of 85 years. Between 1993 and 1995, 22,221 older adults over the age of 65 years died as a result of falling (http://www.cdc.gov). The rate of fall-related deaths increased by 4% from 1995 to 1996 (http://www.nsc.org). Incidence rates for falling range from 0.2 to 0.8 per person annually for community-dwelling older adults, to 2.9 to 3.6 for individuals residing in long-term care facilities (Tideiksaar, 1997). Falls tend to occur within the first few weeks upon entering a nursing home. The reasons sited for these fall-related incidences include unfamiliar environment, medications, the current diagnosis(es), the acuteness of the current diagnosis(es), and immobility or inactivity due to long times sitting or being confined to bed.

Hip fractures cause the greatest morbidity and mortality rates (National Center for Injury Prevention and Control, 1988–1995, 1996; Grisso et al.,

1990). Of the approximately 240,000 hip fractures sustained each year, nearly 80% are sustained by women. It is estimated that upwards of 90% of the hip fractures are a result of falling (Melton, 1988). Hip fractures alone account for $3 billion in direct medical costs each year not including the costs for short- and long-term rehabilitation or for home health care (Norris, 1992). Over half of those older adults who sustain hip fractures that require hospitalization cannot return home or live independently. One-third of these individuals will die within a year following the fall. In addition to hip fractures, distal forearm or wrist fractures are other common fracture sites (Nevitt & Cummings, 1993). Kelsey, Browner, Seeley, Nevitt, and Cummings (1992) postulated that women who are in good health and active, and who have good neuromuscular function but low bone density, tend to sustain distal forearm fractures during falls. Conversely, women who are less healthy and less active, and who have lower neuromuscular functioning and low bone density, are more likely to sustain proximal humerus (hip) fractures. Head trauma (Sattin et al., 1990) and other musculoskeletal injuries may also occur.

Falls produce more than just physical consequences, such as the fear of falling. This fear, obviously, is prevalent in older adults with osteoporosis. Fear of falling can lead to loss of self-confidence to perform routine activities of daily living (ADL) and social isolation (Tinetti & Powell, 1993). Individuals who self-report a fear of falling concurrent with a decrease in activity level are significantly more inclined to be socially isolated and less willing to talk to family or others about falls (Howland et al., 1998).

The cause of falling is multifactorial (Grisso et al., 1991; Tinetti et al., 1994). Individuals with osteoporosis may have a progressive kyphotic posture, which alters the biochemical alignment of the body by shifting the center of gravity more forward. To maintain the head in an upright position, an increased compensation by the neck occurs. However, other factors need to be considered in addition to postural alignment and low bone density. Risk factors for falls also include history of falling, previous fractures, taking four or more medications, visual impairments, lower extremity weakness, balance and gait impairments, and neurologic impairments. Environmental factors, such as carpeting, obstacles, and lighting, also play a prominent role in falls and fall-related injuries. Although many of the falls among community-dwelling older adults occur in and around the home, the data are equivocal as to whether or not more falls and injuries occur inside or outside the home.

Health care professionals can provide fall prevention programs to cohorts of older adults independent of their current living status (e.g., community, residential facility, nursing home, and hospital). Special emphasis should be placed on those individuals who have or are predisposed to osteoporosis. The following six principles need to be considered when developing a fall prevention program:

1.   What causes a fall in one individual may not necessarily cause a fall in another individual.

2.   Falls can lead to a fear of falling as well as a fear of the inability to get back up after a fall has occurred.

3.   Inactivity is a fall risk behavior. Inactivity includes the spectrum from prolonged bed rest to an inactive life (Campbell, Borrie, & Spears, 1989). Older persons with a history of falls with fractures or osteoporosis may almost automatically choose a less active lifestyle to avoid falling. However, inactivity itself may lead to a loss of self-confidence and an increased risk of falling.

4.   Physiologic factors such as muscle and skeletal strength, balance, gait, and reaction time are associated with an increased risk for falling. The risk of falls increases with the number of physiologic risk factors, the number of medications, and the number of functional impairments. These factors are not only important to identify in terms of fall risk and potential fall-related injuries, but they are also important to consider when preventing or reducing the impact of a fall.

5.   A fall prevention program should include a screening component, an education component, and an activity component.

6.   An older adult may not be committed to make the recommended changes in his/her lifestyles or home environment for a variety of social, cultural, financial, or personal reasons.

Generally, fall prevention programs have been custom-designed for specific settings. Therefore, a single reliable and valid fall prevention program does not exist. The elements of a fall prevention program are listed in the section that follows. These elements include a self-report of those factors that may contribute to falls, a balance screen, an educational and activity component, and a follow-up component. The general elements of a program are outlined below and elaborated in an example program, Fall Prevention Program for Community-Dwelling Older Adults. The purpose of any fall prevention program is to inform and motivate older adults to make necessary adaptations to their lifestyles and home environment to reduce the risk for falls. No program can guarantee a reduction in falls if the information is not relevant or they do not actively do their part to reduce their risks.

ELEMENTS OF A FALL PREVENTION PROGRAM

Fall Risk and Balance Screen

A quick assessment is needed to determine if referral to other health care professionals is needed. Items to consider include:

FALL HISTORY

Determine the circumstances surrounding one fall or repeated falls. Fall history can be as simple as asking if the older adult has fallen within the past six months, or may be more comprehensive, i.e., logging the fall(s) in terms of time of day, activity surrounding the fall, location of the fall inside or outside the house.

FEAR OF FALLING INDEX

A simple question is to ask the individual if any reduction in activities has occurred due to a fear of falling. More detailed assessments determine the confidence an individual has performing routine activities. Two measures are the Fear of Falling Index (Tinetti, Richman, & Powell, 1990) and the Activity-Specific Balance Confidence (ABC) Scale (Powell & Myers, 1995).

HEALTH STATUS

Self-report of the individual's perception of their health is a simple question: "How do you perceive your health?" The rating is excellent, good, fair, or poor.

MEDICAL HISTORY

It is important to assess medical history related to any chronic or acute conditions the person has that might contribute to falls. Particular attention should be directed to musculoskeletal disorders, vision, cardiovascular status, cognitive status, and sensation. In addition, the number of medications is ascertained, including prescribed and over-the-counter medications. The use of a mobility aid such as a cane or walker is also noted.

Measure of Physical Performance and Ability to Accomplish Activities of Daily Living

Examples of test batteries that actually measure the functional ability to perform specific physical activities include the following:

- Established Populations for Epidemiology Studies of the Elderly (EPESE) tests balance, walking, and strength (Guralnik et al., 1994).
- Performance Activities of Daily Living (PADL) (Kuriansky & Gurland, 1976) simulates activities of daily living.
- Physical Disability Index (Gerety et al., 1993) includes range of motion, strength, balance, and mobility and is designed for nursing home or frail individuals.
- Physical Performance Test (Reuben & Sie, 1990) includes manual abilities, strength, balance, and mobility.
- Physical Performance and Mobility Examination (Winograd et al., 1994) tests mobility and walking. It is designed for hospitalized patients.

Balance Assessments

Several easy to administer and reliable balance assessments are indicated below. More extensive review of these and additional balance and gait assessments are located elsewhere (Rubenstein, Wieland, & Bernabei, 1995; Studenski & Rigler, 1996).

- Multi-Directional Reach Test (MDRT) (Newton, 1997) measures limits of stability by having the person reach in the forward, right, and left directions and lean backwards. This test is a modification of the Forward Reach (Duncan, Weiner, Chandler, & Studenski, 1990) that only measures reach in the forward direction.

- Timed Up and Go (TUG) (Podsiadlo & Richardson, 1991) times the individual standing from a chair, walking 10 feet, and returning to the original seated position.
- Performance Oriented Mobility Assessment (POMA) (Tinetti, 1986) assesses balance and gait.
- Berg Balance Test (Berg, Wood-Dauphinee, Williams, & Gayton, 1989) assesses balance performance during functional tasks.

Education and Activity

When addressing modifications to lifestyle or the environment, considerations should include cultural, financial, relevance to older adults, and the willingness of individuals to change. Several rather than many suggestions are recommended so as not to overwhelm or frustrate the older adult. Group participation to identify fall risk behavior and ways to modify these behaviors is one strategy to use. Generally, older adults are more willing to change the environment than themselves.

MODIFICATIONS TO ONE'S LIFESTYLE

Suggestions include:

- Wear appropriate clothing and shoes. For example, long bathrobes cause tripping.
- Participate in activity. Appropriate activities include low impact exercises, dancing, gardening, walking, Tai Chi, and other social or physical activities that fit into the lifestyle of the individual. Specific exercises for individuals with osteoporosis are discussed in chapter 5 (Prior, Farr, Chow, & Faulkner, 1996; Henderson, White, & Eisman, 1998).
- Eat healthily. Nutrition is discussed in chapter 4.

HOW TO GET UP FROM THE FLOOR

Older adults need a strategy to get up once a fall has occurred. The strategy may be yelling for help, crawling to a telephone, or getting up alone (see Table 9.1).

TABLE 9.1 Teaching Community-Dwelling Older Adults to Get Up from the Floor

The following is a general instruction sheet. Personal experience or other hints are encouraged to make the talk appropriate to the audience.

Many older adults have a fear of falling and have a great fear of being unable to get up once a fall has occurred. It is important that older persons know how to get up from the floor. It is particularly important for those individuals who live alone. The longer a person remains on the floor following a fall, the greater the chances for secondary complications resulting from lying there. It is a given that everyone falls.

Before the person attempts to get up, determine if someone is available to assist. If the person is living with someone, it is better to call for assistance, even if it means waking the person up. The fall may have caused an injury or badly shaken the person. In all cases the key is to move slowly, remain calm, and run through your mind the next step in getting up.

First, check to see if anything is broken; that is, does the bone feel broken, or does it just really hurt a lot? Generally, broken bones are associated with severe pain. If the person is living alone and believes that something is broken, the person needs to move on the floor to reach a telephone. This is done slowly.

Ask the audience, how would they get up from the floor if they have fallen. If the floor is clean (always bring a floor covering) lay down and have the group problem solve how you would get up. This way they see the demonstration as well as being actively involved by providing hints. (Most groups enjoy this and will provide additional hints.)

The steps include moving along the floor to a sturdy chair that will not move, the sofa, or some other fixed support (not a bathroom sink because it could pull away from the wall).

- Moving can occur by pulling oneself along, crawling, or scooting.
- Get into a side-sitting position. Once in this position, pause a second to get your bearings (orient yourself and catch your breath).
- Kneel with support of the chair, sofa, etc. Once in this position, pause a second to get your bearings (orient yourself and catch your breath).
- Use the stronger knee to push yourself into the chair or sofa. Putting the forearms on the chair or sofa seat also helps to get some leverage. Once in this position, pause a second to get your bearings (orient yourself and catch your breath).

It is important to emphasize doing this slowly and not impulsively just because the person is embarrassed that a fall occurred. Once sitting in a chair or on the sofa, take time to calm down, catch your breath, and decide the next course of action. That is, do I need to call a friend, neighbor, relative, the ambulance, or 911 for help? Do I just need to talk to someone for assurance?

For those individuals who may be reluctant to learn to get up because of fear or anxiety, or because they do not feel that they have the physical capability to get up, then other strategies are needed. For example, some individuals may be able to afford some type of alarm system. For all people, recommend a buddy system that is having someone call at least once a day. Also, recommend placing the telephone in easy reach and not attached to a kitchen wall where one has to stand to use it. Have a relative give the person a portable telephone for Christmas or another holiday.

MODIFICATIONS TO THE ENVIRONMENT

Making the living space safe can best be achieved by providing a room-by-room assessment or commonalties (lighting, flooring, and stairs). Recommendations for environmental modifications should take into account financial constraints.

IDENTIFY RESOURCES

Once modifications are recommended, it is helpful to provide location of resources. These resources may include retired older persons with skills to help other seniors, projects by vocational schools or professional organizations, local agencies that provide health care or social services, health or social service professionals, and computer searches on the Web. Lastly, gifts to give the older adult include help aids (e.g., grabbers, a portable telephone, a flashlight, and night lights).

Follow-Up

Providing a follow-up program is extremely helpful to answer questions older adults may have regarding the educational program, or to identify sources of assistance to correct environmental hazards. In addition, the follow-up session provides an opportunity to determine why the individual is not compliant, and then to develop an appropriate revision of strategies.

FALL PREVENTION PROGRAM FOR COMMUNITY-DWELLING OLDER ADULTS

The following program is an example of a specific fall prevention program that was developed using the information provided above. The Fall Prevention Program for Community-Dwelling Older Adults can be modified based on the discipline of the participating professionals, the time available for such a program, and the needs of the community receiving the program. Additionally, the program can be modified for use in other settings and with other cohorts of older adults. The Fall Prevention Program can be translated for those older adults whose first language is not English. The self-assessment portion can be read to the older adult who has visual or reading impairments. The following are components of a Fall Prevention Program developed by the author (Newton, 1998).

Fall Risk Assessment

1. Do you _____ live alone or _____ with others?
2. Have you fallen in the past 6 months? _____
3. In the past 5 years, have you fallen and broken a bone? _____
   If so where? _____
4. Medical history: Check or circle all those that apply to you.
   _____ Number of medications (it is ideal to have them show you the medications that they take)
   _____ Use a mobility aid _____ none _____ cane _____ walker
   _____ Heart problems (hypertension, heart attack or other heart problems, Peripheral Vascular Disease)
   _____ Respiratory problems (difficulty breathing, emphysema, allergies)
   _____ Visual problems (wears glasses, glaucoma, or other visual impairments)
   _____ Hearing problems (difficulty hearing, wear a hearing aid)
   _____ Poor sensation (feeling) in the feet
   _____ Musculoskeletal problems (arthritis, osteoporosis, muscle cramps)
   _____ Diabetes
   _____ Dizziness or an unsteady feeling
5. How do you rate your health?_____ Excellent _____ Good _____ Fair _____ Poor
6. Do you have a fear of falling? If so, has the fear changed your activity level (lifestyle)?
   _____ Not Afraid
   _____ Afraid but have not changed my activity level (lifestyle)
   _____ Afraid and have changed my activity (lifestyle)

Balance Assessment

1. Multi-Directional Reach Test
2. Timed Up and Go

3. A spotter assists with all balance testing. As time permits, the Berg Balance Test or other balance test can be administered.

Education

1. Modification of lifestyle. Items can include those listed below. Time is permitted for discussion.
    Wash glasses when brushing teeth so both are clean.
    Wear appropriate shoes and clothing.
    Refrain from sharing medications. "Brown bag" all medications and take them to the pharmacist or primary physician to check for drug interactions or those medications that are no longer required.
2. Demonstrate how to get up after a fall and include group discussion as to how they would get up.
3. Environmental risk factors, such as:
    Have someone change light bulbs that are burned out.
    Provide a checklist of no more than 10 items for environmental change. The items range from those that can be done quickly and without cost to those that are more costly and require a repairman.
    Identify local resources to help with repairs, donations.

Activities

Discuss with the group those activities that are appropriate for individuals with osteoporosis. Activities range from low impact exercises to Tai Chi, square dancing, dancing, social activities, and so on.

Other Activities

Pass out fall prevention brochures and other relevant brochures.

A drawing for a prize for participation. Prizes could include a health aid or other item related to safety and prevention.

Follow-Up

One month after the program the health care professional can meet with the group to discuss their accomplishments and to complete a questionnaire.

The questionnaire includes items such as falls in the past month as well as benefits of the program. The items on the checklist can be modified into a questionnaire to determine benefits of the fall prevention program in terms of modifications made to the person's lifestyle or home environment. The three examples that follow attempt to determine if the modification was made, and if not, was the reason due to relevance of the item, financial, or that the individual is not yet willing to make change.

YES	NO	
_____	_____	I installed grab bars.
_____	_____	I already had them.
_____	_____	They cost too much.
_____	_____	No one could install them.
_____	_____	I do not think they are necessary.

YES	NO	
_____	_____	I have been doing the low impact activity program at home.
_____	_____	I do not find them helpful.
_____	_____	I would prefer to do my normal routine activity such as walking.
_____	_____	They interfere with my daily routine.
_____	_____	I lost the sheet.
_____	_____	I will start doing them tomorrow.

YES	NO	
_____	_____	Did you fall in the past month?
_____	_____	If you fell, did you find the information on getting up helpful?
_____	_____	If you have not fallen, did you find the information on getting up helpful?

In summary, falls can be reduced by a conscious effort on the part of all health care and social service professionals and older adults, perhaps with the help of their families and/or friends. Fall prevention programs can be implemented in nursing homes or as part of community activity programs. If one older adult can reduce the risk of falls, then the quality of life for that individual will be greatly improved. And if health-related professionals, individually or across disciplines, can institute fall prevention programs in their facilities and in their communities, then the number of falls and fall-related injuries will significantly decrease. Thus, older adults can enjoy a healthier and better quality of life as they move into the 21st century.

REFERENCES

Berg, K., Wood-Dauphinee, S., Williams, J., & Gayton, D. (1989). Measuring balance in the elderly: Preliminary development of an instrument. *Physiotherapy Canada, 41,* 304–311.

Campbell, A. J., Borrie, M. J., & Spears, G. F. (1989). Risk factors for falls in a community-based prospective study of people 70 years and older. *Journal of Gerontology, 44,* M112–M117.

Duncan, P. W., Weiner, D. K., Chandler, J., & Studenski, S. (1990). Functional reach: A new clinical measure of balance. *Journal of Gerontology, 45,* M192–M197.

Gerety, M. B., Mulrow, C. D., Tuley, M. R., Hazuda, H. P., Lichtenstein, M. J., Bohannon, R., Kanten, D. N., O'Neil, M. B., & Gorton, A. (1993). Development and validation of a physical performance instrument for the functionally impaired elderly: The physical disability index (PDI). *Journal of Gerontology, 48,* M33–M38.

Grisso, J. A., Swartz, D. F., Wishner, A. R., Weene, B., Holmes, J. H., & Sutton, R. L. (1990). Injuries in an elderly inner-city population. *Journal of the American Geriatrics Society, 38,* 1326–1331.

Grisso, J. A., Kelsey, J. L., Strom, B. L., Chiu, G. Y., Maislin, G., O'Brien, L. A., Hoffman, S., & Kaplan, F. (1991). Risk factors for falls as a cause of hip fracture in women: The northeast hip fracture study group. *New England Journal of Medicine, 324,* 1326–1331.

Guralnik, J. M., Simonsick, E. M., Ferrucci, L., Glynn, R. J., Berkman, L. F., Blazer, D. G., Scherr, P. A., & Wallace, R. B. (1994). A short physical performance battery assessing lower extremity function: Association with self-reported disability and prediction of mortality and nursing home admission. *Journal of Gerontology, 49,* M85–M94.

Henderson, N., White, C., & Eisman, J. (1998). The roles of exercise and fall risk reduction in the prevention of osteoporosis. *Endocrinology and Metabolism Clinics of North America, 27,* 369–387.

Howland, J., Lachman, M. E., Peterson, E. W., Cote, J., Kasten, L., & Jette, A. (1998). Covariates of falling and associated activity curtailment. *Gerontologist, 38,* 549–555.

Kelsey, J. L., Browner, W. S., Seeley, D. G., Nevitt, M. C., & Cummings, S. R. (1992). Risk factors for fractures of the distal forearm and proximal humerus: The study of osteoporotic fractures research group. *American Journal of Epidemiology, 135,* 477–489.

Kuriansky, J., & Gurland, B. (1976). The performance test of activities of daily living. *International Journal of Aging and Human Development, 7,* 343–352.

Melton, L. J. III. (1988). Epidemiology of fractures. In B. Riggs & L. Melton (Eds.), *Osteoporosis: Etiology, diagnosis and management* (pp. 133–154). New York: Raven.

National Center for Injury Prevention and Control (1988–1994, 1996). *National Survey of Injury Mortality Data*. Atlanta, GA: Centers for Disease Control and Prevention.

Nevitt, M., & Cummings, S. (1993). Type of fall and risk of hip and wrist fractures: The study of osteoporotic fractures. *Journal of the American Geriatrics Society, 42*, 909.

Newton, R. A. (1997). Balance screening of an inner city older adult population. *Archives of Physiological Medicine and Rehabilitation, 78*, 587–591.

Norris, R. J. (1992). Medical costs of osteoporosis. *Bone, 13*(Suppl. 2), S11–16.

Podsiadlo, D., & Richardson, S. (1991). The timed "Up & Go": A test of basic functional mobility for frail elderly persons. *Journal of the American Geriatrics Society, 39*, 142–148.

Powell, L. E., & Myers, A. M. (1995). The activities-specific balance confidence (ABC) scale. *Journal of Gerontology. Series A, Biological Sciences & Medical Sciences, 50A*, M28–M34.

Prior, J., Farr, S., Chow, R., & Faulkner, R. (1996). Physical activity as therapy for osteoporosis. *Canadian Medical Association Journal, 155*, 940–944.

Reuben, D., & Sie, A. (1990). An objective measure of physical function of elderly patients: The physical performance test. *Journal of the American Geriatrics Society, 38*, 1105–1112.

Rubenstein, L. Z., Wieland, D., & Bernabei, R. (1995). Geriatric assessment technology: The state of the art. *Aging, 7*, 157–158.

Sattin, R. W., Huber D. A. L., DeVito, C. A., Rodriguez, J. G., Ros, A., Bacchelli, S., Stevens, J. A., & Waxweiller, R. J. (1990). The incidence of fall injury events among elderly in a defined population. *American Journal of Epidemiology, 131*, 1028–1037.

Studenski, S. C., & Rigler, S. K. (1996). Clinical overview of instability in the elderly. *Clinics in Geriatric Medicine, 12*, 679–688.

Tideiksaar, R. (1997). *Falling in old age: Prevention and management* (2nd ed.). New York: Springer.

Tinetti, M. E. (1986). Performance-oriented assessment of mobility problems in elderly patients. *Journal of the American Geriatrics Society, 34*, 119–126.

Tinetti, M. E., Baker, D. I., McAvay, G., Claus, E. B., Garrett, P., Gottschalk, M., Koch, M. L., Trainor, K., & Horwitz, R. I. (1994). A multifactorial intervention to reduce the risk of falling among elderly people living in the community. *New England Journal of Medicine, 331*, 821–827.

Tinetti, M. E., Richman, D., & Powell, L. (1990). Falls efficacy as a measure of fear of falling. *Journal of Gerontology, 45*, P239–P243.

Tinetti, M. E., & Powell, L. (1993). Fear of falling and low self-efficacy: A case of dependence in elderly persons. *Journal of Gerontology, 48*(Special Issue), 35–38.

Tinetti, M. E., Speechley, M., & Ginter, S. (1998). Risk factors for falls among elderly persons living in the community. *New England Journal of Medicine, 319*, 1701–1707.

Winograd, C. H., Lemsky, C. M., Nevitt, M. C., Nordstrom, T. M., Stewart, A. L., Miller, C. J., & Bloch, D. A. (1994). Development of a physical performance and mobility examination. *Journal of the American Geriatrics Society, 42,* 743–749.

10

Relief of Pain

Sarah Hall Gueldner, Eric D. Newman, Phil Hanus, and Gail B. Shirk

> Pain management is a moral imperative for those in the profession of healing.
>
> —T. Borneman and B. R. Ferrell

Although the onset of osteoporosis is silent, most persons with osteoporosis eventually experience the phenomenon of pain to some degree. Although the classic recurrent, nontrauma-associated vertebral fractures may occur with a surprising absence of pain, hip fractures precipitated by falls are characteristically accompanied by excruciating pain. Additionally, chronic pain related to multiple vertebral compression fractures is almost certain to appear in the later stages of osteoporosis. In fact, osteoporosis was one of the three most commonly reported diagnoses in geriatric patients who report chronic pain (Cutler, Fishbain, Rosomoff, & Rosomoff, 1994). Anecdotal data indicate that many persons with osteoporosis have lived with chronic pain so long that they have become accustomed to it and accept it as just a necessary and constant part of their lives. However, in spite of compelling evidence that most persons with osteoporosis experience pain, pain management is seldom mentioned as a part of the care plan for osteoporosis.

MUST ELDERS "GRIN AND BEAR IT?"

Because the painful effects of osteoporosis usually manifest in older adults, effective pain management does pose a particular challenge. The possibility of adverse interaction of pain relievers with drugs being taken for coexisting conditions increases with age; and opioids, the most commonly used pain relievers, are known for their interaction with other drugs. Opioids are also associated with a high incidence of other untoward effects, including constipation, ileus, confusion, sedation, and in some instances respiratory depression. Additionally, a large percentage of patients who sustain hip fractures become confused or disoriented, making it even more difficult to assess and treat their pain.

Perhaps for the reasons just listed, undertreatment of the elderly in general has been confirmed in the literature (Short, Burnett, Egbert, & Parks, 1990). Even in the absence of any evidence that they experience diminished pain intensity or have higher tolerance to pain, research findings have shown that elders tend to be treated less aggressively than younger patients. For instance, in a study of 97 elderly patients by Ferrell and Ferrell (1995), 71% had at least one pain complaint, 34% described continuous pain, and 66% described intermittent pain. Although most (84%) had physician's orders, only 15% had received medication for pain within the past 24 hours. The problem of undertreatment is no doubt exacerbated by common problems associated with aging, including memory or sensory impairment and delayed metabolism of medications. Selected barriers to effective pain management in elders are listed in Table 10.1.

Inadequate pain management has recently come under serious scrutiny by health care professionals from across disciplines and is no longer acceptable under any circumstances. Pain relief is increasingly being described as an ethical issue and is considered a moral imperative for those in the profession of healing. The International Association for the Study of Pain (IASP) has led a major campaign to raise the profile of pain and its management through its journal, *Pain,* and the triennial congresses on pain. A special-interest group for the study of pain in older persons has been formed within this group, and pain in older persons will be featured at future congresses (Helme et al., 1996). Leaders of this organization have joined with other

TABLE 10.1 **Barriers to Pain Management in Elders**

- Elders are more susceptible to medication side effects, making pain management more difficult
- Fear of addiction on the part of both the professional and the patient
- A lack of pain assessment instruments with established validity and reliability for use with elderly populations
- Existing misconceptions, such as:

  1. Pain is "an expected part of aging"; elders feel they should be able to "tough it out."
  2. Older patients do not experience the same intensity of pain as their younger counterparts
  3. Older patients have a higher tolerance for pain than younger persons
  4. Older persons cannot tolerate opioids
  5. Persons with cognitive impairment cannot be adequately assessed for pain.

Note. From Egbert (1996); Forman (1996); Parmelee, Smith, & Katz (1993); Stein & Ferrell (1996).

health care groups, such as nurses, in a campaign to add pain as the "fifth vital sign," along with pulse, respiration, blood pressure, and temperature.

PAIN ASSESSMENT

In the best of worlds, the initial evaluation of pain starts with a thorough medical history and physical examination. It also includes an in-depth review of the nature, intensity, and location of the pain (including patient-initiated descriptors), identification of any persistent noxious stimuli, and patterns of relief that have helped in the past. Additionally, assessment should include the impact of the pain on movement/function, sleep, and mood. Psychosocial aspects of the evaluation focus on behavioral responses to the pain, adjustments to impairment and disability, motivational factors, and the impact of the pain on the patient's social support system (Grabois, 1988). Because pain and depression are often entwined, it is recommended that a measure of depression be included as a regular part of the assessment of chronic pain. A number of reliable paper-and-pencil questionnaires are available, including the McGill Pain Questionnaire (MPQ) (McGuire, 1988), the Short Form of the McGill Pain Questionnaire (SF-MPQ) (Melzack, 1987), the visual analogue scale for pain (VASP) (Gift, 1989; McGuire, 1988; Miller & Perry, 1990; Woodforde & Merskey, 1972a, 1972b), and the verbal descriptor scale (VDS) (McGuire, 1988).

No   Pain as
Pain   ─────────────────────────   Bad as It
                                                      Can Be

FIGURE 10.1   Visual Analogue Scale for Pain (VASP).

Note: Adapted from "Some relationships between subjective measures of pain," by J. M. Woodforde & H. Merskey, 1972, in *Journal of Psychosomatic Research, 16*, pp. 173–178. "Personality traits of patients with chronic pain," by J. M. Woodforde and H. Meskey, 1972, *Journal of Psychosomatic Research, 16*, pp. 167–172.

However, time or the patient's condition may not permit such a comprehensive pain assessment. The simplest measure of the intensity of acute pain is a visual analogue scale, which consists of a 100-mm line labeled "no pain" at the left end of the line and "pain as bad as it possibly could be" at the other end (Egbert, 1996; Woodforde & Merskey, 1971, 1972). A graphic representation of the visual analogue scale is provided in Figure 10.1. The patient should be asked more than once about his or her pain, and the clinician should look for and record nonverbal behaviors such as facial grimaces, agitation, or unusually quiet behaviors (Egbert, 1996). It is especially important that pain be assessed on a regular basis to monitor the effectiveness of the pain-management program.

THERAPEUTIC OPTIONS FOR MANAGING PAIN

Most pain-management protocols used today involve pharmaceutical products, at least in part. It is important to be aware that elders are more susceptible to medication side effects than younger persons, and because of comorbid conditions, they are likely to be taking multiple medications. Table 10.2 illustrates the comorbidity issue, highlighting one group of commonly prescribed analgesics, nonsteroidal antiinflammatory drugs (NSAIDs), and other conventional drugs/drug classifications used with the elderly.

It is also important to realize that elders are prone to polyanalgesia, and that 72% of the medications they take are obtained without prescription by purchasing over the counter, borrowing from friends or relatives, or relying on folk remedies (Chrischilles, Lemke, Wallace, & Drube, 1990). The following section will serve as a review and update of principles of

TABLE 10.2 Comparison of Drug Interactions Reported for Selected NSAIDs

	Celecoxib (Celebrex)	Etodolac (Lodine)	Ibuprofen (Motrin, Advil, Nuprin)	Nabumetone (Relafen)	Naproxen (Naprosyn)
ACEI	X*	✓	✓	✓	✓
Diuretics ♥	X*	✓	X	X	X
Aspirin	X	X	X	X	X
Fluconazole	X				
Lithium	X	X	X	✓	X
Methotrexate		X	X	✓	X
Warfarin		X	X	✓	✓
Antacids	X	X			
Cyclosporine		X	✓	✓	✓
Digoxin		X			
Beta-blockers		✓	✓	✓	✓

X = drug interaction listed in the FDA-approved product labeling.

✓ = drug interaction listed in other compendiums or drug-interaction textbooks.

* = based on experience with NSAIDs not celecoxib, but included in the celecoxib product labeling.

♥ = patients with renal dysfunction where prostaglandin production is important to maintain renal perfusion.

Note: Compiled by the Penn State Geisinger Health System Formulary Steering Committee (1999). COX-2 selective inhibitors: Celecoxib (Celebrex®) and Rofecoxib (Vioxx®). *Penn State Geisinger Health System Pharmacy and Therapeutics Review.* Danville, PA: Penn State Geisinger Health System. Adapted from Beaird, S., Djonisi, M. S., Sasich, L. (1999). Etodolac (drug evaluation). In C. R. Gelman, B. H. Rumack, & T. A. Hutchison (Eds.), *DRUGDEX® System.* Englewood, CO: MICROMEDEX, Inc. Benz, J. & DRUGDEX® Editorial Staff. (1999). Nabumetone (drug evaluation). In C. R. Gelman, B. H. Rumack, & T. A. Hutchison (Eds.), *DRUGDEX® System.* Englewood, CO: MICROMEDEX, Inc. Cohon, M. S., Hoffman, R., Salter, F. J., et al. (1999). Ibuprofen (drug evaluation). In C. R. Gelman, B. H. Rumack, & T. A. Hutchison (Eds.), *DRUGDEX® System.* Englewood, CO: MICROMEDEX, Inc. Del Favero, A., Wang, I. H., Wenke, L. A., & DRUGDEX® Editorial Staff. (1999). Naproxen (drug evaluation). In C. R. Gelman, B. H. Rumack, & T. A. Hutchison (Eds.), *DRUGDEX® System.* Englewood, CO: MICROMEDEX, Inc. DRUGDEX® Editorial Staff. (1999). Celecoxib (drug evaluation). In C. R. Gelman, B. H. Rumack, & T. A. Hutchison (Eds.), *DRUGDEX® System.* Englewood, CO: MICROMEDEX, Inc.

pharmaceutical relief of acute and chronic pain in elders. Specific information about pharmaceutical products and dosage is available in traditional sources and will not be repeated in this discussion. Instead, the following space will be used to outline specific advantages and disadvantages of analgesic drugs commonly used to relieve pain in elders. Two categories, nonsteroidal antiinflammatory drugs and opioids, will be reviewed. Selected nonpharmaceutical strategies for relieving pain also will be reviewed.

NONSTEROIDAL ANTIINFLAMMATORY DRUGS

Nonsteroidal antiinflammatory drugs offer an alternative to narcotics for moderate to moderately severe pain and may be combined with opioids to enhance analgesia. Drugs in this category that are not recommended for use with elders include tolmetin (Tolectin), piroxicam (Feldene), meclofenamate (Meclomen), fenoprofen (Nalfon), and aspirin, except for low-dose prophylaxis. Parenteral NSAIDs, such as ketorolac (Toradol), have been used for postoperative pain, both to spare narcotics and as the sole analgesic agents. However, NSAIDs cannot generally be used alone to effectively control pain after major surgery (Smallman, Powell, Ewart, & Morgan, 1992). Intramuscular (IM) or intravenous (IV) ketorolac or IV diclofenac have been found to reduce narcotic requirements by 50%–75% (Egbert, 1996; Smallman et al., 1992). Likewise, research has shown that a single dose of controlled-release indomethacin or oral ibuprofen preoperatively can decrease pain and reduce narcotic use postoperatively (Rowe, Goodwin, & Miller, 1992).

NSAIDs may also be used to reduce unwanted side effects of analgesia. For instance, use of IM ketorolac instead of IM meperidine was shown to reduce time to unassisted walking, first bowel movement, urinary retention, and hypoventilation (Stahlgren et al., 1993). A major concern with the use of NSAIDs in frail elders is acute renal failure (Stein & Ferrell, 1996), and for this reason they should be used cautiously and always accompanied with sufficient hydration.

Postoperative bleeding is another important issue with this class of medication. NSAIDs produce platelet inhibition that may increase postoperative bleeding and, more important, increase bleeding when coupled with prophylactic anticoagulants used to prevent deep vein thrombosis. It is important for the clinician to be mindful of these adverse effects and to take steps to prevent further complications for the elderly client.

An important concern with chronic NSAID use is gastrointestinal (GI) bleeding. Although only a small proportion of NSAID users develop ulcers, the odds increase significantly in patients over age 55. Risk factors for serious gastrointestinal complications have been examined using the ARAMIS database (Fries, Williams, Bloch, & Michel, 1991). A scoring system was developed that allows placement of a patient in a higher risk group.

Variables important in this risk stratification include age, prior NSAID-related gastrointestinal problem, disability level, NSAID dose, and current prednisone use. Other factors that may increase the risk of NSAID-induced gastrointestinal damage include (a) gender—elderly females may be more likely to experience an NSAID-associated ulcer, and (b) previous history of peptic ulcer disease and *H. pylori* (Fries et al., 1991; Silverstein et al., 1995).

NSAID-associated ulcers do not correlate well with pain, perhaps because the analgesic action of NSAIDs may mask the ulcer pain (Smith, 1995). Many patients who take NSAIDs take them for chronic pain conditions. Therefore, their perception of pain may be changed, and they may tend to ignore ulcer symptoms. The elderly appear to be predisposed to silent ulcers; therefore, complications such as gastrointestinal bleeding and perforation are more likely to develop without symptoms. It is not unusual to find silent perforations or gastroduodenal ulcerations in asymptomatic individuals (Smith, 1995). It is important to note that the addition of usual doses of H_2 blockers or proton pump inhibitors may mask ulcer pain but do not prevent gastric ulcers (Ehsanullah, Page, Tildesley, & Wood, 1988; Robinson et al., 1989).

A new generation of NSAIDs, known as the cyclooxygenase-2 (COX-2) inhibitors, provide relief equal to standard NSAIDs but with a marked reduction in endoscopic gastric erosions and ulcerations. It is believed that this will also translate into a lower incidence of severe clinical gastrointestinal events (bleeding, perforation, and death). Standard NSAIDs exhibit their beneficial effects (reduction in inflammation and pain) by blocking the COX-2 pathway and their side effects (gastrointestinal, platelet dysfunction) by blocking the COX-1 (cyclooxygenase-1) pathway. By blocking COX-2 selectively, this new generation, which includes medications such as rofecoxib (Vioxx) and celecoxib (Celebrex), appears to provide an added safety margin in high-risk patients who need an NSAID. Currently, only Vioxx is approved for pain control. Both medications should be avoided in patients with significant renal disease.

OPIOIDS

Opioids exert their effect through receptor binding in the central nervous system because of their resemblance to endogenously produced opioids (endorphins) that act throughout the nervous system. The most often used are opioids agonists, which include propoxyphene, codeine, oxycodone, hydrocodone, morphine, hydromorphone, meperidine, methadone, fentanyl, tramadol, and levorphanol (Forman, 1996). Even though fewer than 1% of those taking opioids become addicted (McCaffery & Beebe, 1989), professionals still tend to think of them as addicting and thus tend to prescribe them sparingly. It is true that when a person receives opioids for a period of time, he or she will develop dependence. If the opioid is abruptly discontinued, the person will have symptoms that resemble the withdrawal symptoms that addicts experience (sweats, abdominal cramps, malaise, and anxiety). However, unlike the addict, the normal person will not develop a craving for opioids. Withdrawal symptoms can be eliminated by tapering the opioid dosage by 25% each day until the desired dose is reached, or until the drug is finally discontinued (Forman, 1996). For unknown reasons, opioid tolerance develops and imposes a gradual decrease in analgesic effect over time. This observed tolerance is no different in elders than in younger populations (Brescia, 1987).

Another category of drugs to consider, although not used as often for chronic pain, is the opioid partial agonists. Drugs such as Stadol, Talwin, and Nubain are included in this category. More commonly used to manage acute pain, these agents have no advantages over narcotics for treatment of chronic pain and, when taken orally, have poor efficacy. Psychotomimetic side effects such as hallucinations are also of some concern with these agents, although Nubain reportedly induces much less untoward psychotic effects than Stadol or Talwin (Koo, 1995). For these reasons, this class of drugs would not be recommended as first-line therapy in the elderly for treatment of chronic pain secondary to osteoporosis.

Opioids Recommended for Use in Older Adults

Oxycodone is considered to be a weak opioid but is almost equal to morphine when given orally (Forman, 1996). Morphine and hydromorphone are better for postoperative use than meperidine, because they have a greater benefit to risk with regard to pain relief and toxic side effects (Forman, 1996). Oxycodone, morphine, hydromorphone, and fentanyl are appropriate and can usually achieve satisfactory analgesia in both acute and chronic pain management in the elderly persons (Forman, 1996). Codeine, oxycodone, and hydrocodone are generally available in combination with aspirin or acetaminophen and are used for pain that is no longer responsive to other agents such as NSAIDS. However, dosage is limited by the toxicity of the accompanying agent; aspirin increases the risk of GI bleeding and chronic administration of acetaminophen in excess of 5 gm per day has been associated with hepatic enzyme changes. For this reason it is best to use these opioids alone or seek another opioid (Forman, 1996; Koo, 1995).

Morphine has the most cumulative clinical testing and experience (Forman, 1996). Both morphine and hydromorphone can be taken orally, with no difference in effect in the elderly, although oral doses are higher because of poor absorption (Baillie, Bateman, Coates, & Woodhouse, 1989; Hays et al., 1994). Epidural delivery of opioids may bypass some of the unwanted effects of opioids (e.g., somnolence and constipation) (Forman, 1996) but has a higher reported incidence of respiratory depression (Gustafsson, Schildt, & Jacobsen, 1982). Morphine and hydromorphone (Dilaudid) are reliable and effective for use with patient-controlled analgesia (PCA) (Egbert, Parks, Short, & Burnett, 1990; Forman, 1996).

Opioids to Be Used with Caution When Treating Chronic Pain in Elders

Methadone, propoxyphene, and meperidine have metabolites that produce central nervous system toxicity. This occurs when repeated, high doses are used or when used in patients with significant renal dysfunction. For example, one meperidine metabolite, normeperidine, will accumulate in patients with decreased renal clearance and may produce twitching and eventual seizure activity from its excitatory effects (Egbert, 1996). Methadone and levorphanol have longer half-lives than morphine or hydromorphone. Drugs with longer half-lives should be titrated carefully, especially in the elderly population. Fentanyl is not available orally, and transdermal delivery rate may be markedly higher in elders, accompanied by respiratory depression, nausea, and pruritus (Holdsworth, Forman, & Nystrom, 1994).

Unwanted Effects of Opioids

Respiratory depression (because of decreased sensitivity of the central respiratory system centers to CO_2) is the most serious side effect of opioids (Egbert, 1996). Nausea and constipation are the two most often encountered unwanted effects of opioid administration. Other bothersome side effects, particularly noted in elders, include vivid nightmares, myoclonic movements, and overwhelming somnolence. Somnolence may be offset by drinking coffee in the morning, and an antihistamine such as Meclizine may be given the first 3 days to control nausea. Simple bulk laxatives will not be sufficient to eliminate constipation. Instead, bowel-stimulating agents, such as a senna preparation, bisacodyl, or casanthranol with docusate, should be given to prevent constipation. If constipation persists, magnesium citrate or enemas may be necessary. Because clearance of opioids may be decreased in the elderly because of compromised hepatic or renal function, dosing consultations are recommended.

Methods of Delivery

If IM narcotics are used, it is recommended that injections be scheduled rather than given on a prn basis. Oral morphine is an effective alternative if the patient is able to take oral medications; 60 mg of oral morphine is equivalent to 10 mg parenteral (Inturrisi, 1989). Intravenous patient-controlled analgesia (IV-PAC) was found to be more effective than "as needed" IM injections (Boulanger et al., 1993) and was less often associated with respiratory depression than with epidural or IM delivery of analgesia (Benzon et al., 1993). Epidural methadone (Dolophine) has been effective in patients too frail to undergo surgery for proximal femoral fractures (Nyska, Shapira, Klin, Drenger, & Margulies, 1989), but is associated with increased risk of respiratory depression (Weller, Rosenblum, Conard, & Gross, 1991) and urinary retention (Walts, Kaufman, Moreland, & Weiskopf, 1985).

NONPHARMACEUTICAL MODALITIES

Given the many problems associated with medications in the elderly, non-pharmaceutical strategies provide an important alternative approach for either managing their pain or complementing pharmaceutical measures. Heat and cold applications are the most commonly used physical modalities of pain relief. Some persons with osteoporotic pain have also gained satisfactory relief from Transcutaneous Electrical Nerve Stimulation (TENS) (Nguyen, 1996). In fact, there is growing consensus that this modality warrants a trial in most pain conditions irrespective of age because it is safe and of great benefit for some individuals. Helme et al. (1996) warn that a 20-

minute TENS application on two occasions in a consulting room does not provide an adequate trial and suggest that a more suitable trial would be to use TENS for up to 6 hours per day over a 2-week period.

Orthotic devices such as braces to support the back or torso may also provide a measure of pain relief by helping to maintain desirable posture or immobilize the site of pain, thus promoting healing, improving alignment, and assisting function. Considerable success has been reported in the use of spinal orthotic devices to relieve the pain of vertebral compression fractures. Graded exercise programs are also recommended to strengthen muscles and decrease pain resulting from improper alignment and maladaptive movement patterns.

Cognitive Behavioral Therapies

Biofeedback techniques have also been useful in the management of chronic pain. Relaxation techniques such as deep-muscle relaxation, meditation, and self-hypnosis may also be useful in the management of chronic pain by increasing tolerance to pain. However, some believe that cognitive behavioral modification techniques are less effective in older persons than in younger groups, based on speculations that elders may be less likely to have a psychologic contribution to their pain experience (Portenoy & Farkash, 1988).

Nguyen (1996) advocates the interdisciplinary team approach to pain management in elders, arguing that the psychosocial context of pain may be more important in elderly persons than in younger patients (Harkins & Price, 1987). The typical core team of such a pain-management program includes the physician, clinical psychologist, rehabilitation nurse, physical therapist, occupational therapist, and social worker. Others, such as an anesthesiologist, a psychiatrist, and an alternative healer may also be involved.

PAIN FROM COMPRESSION FRACTURE

One third of women over the age of 65 will have vertebral fracture. Conservative management is followed in the absence of neurologic symptoms. If accompanied by pain, opioid analgesics may be used during the acute phase, always with careful attention to bowel patterns, because ileus is a common complication. Calcitonin has also been shown to offer some relief of pain in acute vertebral compression fractures, though the mechanism is not fully understood.

Several studies support the rapid onset and strong analgesic effect of calcitonin on patients with acute vertebral fractures secondary to osteoporosis (Kapuscinski, Talalaj, Borowicz, Marcinowska-Suchowierska, & Brzozowski, 1996; Lyritis et al., 1997; Maksymowych, 1998). In the findings of his meta-analysis, Maksymowych (1998) concluded that after introduction of calcitonin, pain relief occurred within the first 2 weeks, could continue for 4 months, and might occur if treatment were instituted any time within the first year after fracture. He determined that calcitonin in a dose of 50 IU to 100 IU daily, given subcutaneously or intranasally, should be offered to all patients with serious pain related to acute vertebral fractures for symptom relief and to facilitate mobilization.

The person with compression fracture is initially confined to bed rest with cold applications to reduce pain and swelling. Heat therapy and gentle massage may also be useful in alleviating muscle spasms, and TENS application is useful in most cases. However, there is overwhelming evidence that prolonged immobilization has devastating consequences in the elderly (Kottke & Lehmann, 1990), so within a few days the patient should be helped to engage in 10-minute sessions of sitting and walking each hour during the regular daytime hours. The patient should be taught to avoid flexion and kyphotic posture, as these movements could cause additional wedging deformities and lead to new compression fractures. They should also be advised to wear low-heeled and soft-soled shoes to cushion some of the impact on the spine during ambulation. Spinal orthoses may be applied to provide extrinsic support if needed (Nguyen, 1996).

MANAGEMENT OF POSTOPERATIVE PAIN FOLLOWING HIP FRACTURE

Inadequate management of postoperative pain is common among elders. However, as mentioned earlier, management of postoperative pain in elders (e.g., following hip fractures) is fraught with potential complications. Elders are more susceptible to medication side effects than younger populations. The clinicians working with individuals who have surgery following osteoporotic hip fracture must constantly balance these competing considerations. For instance, NSAIDs cause fatal peptic ulcers more often in elders than in younger persons. Likewise, transient apnea and periodic breathing are more common after narcotics, and epidural opioids more frequently produce delayed respiratory depression (Brown, 1985). Postoperative pain management in elders is also complicated by the high incidence of postoperative delirium and preexisting dementia. It is estimated that up to 60% of frail elders experience delirium after femoral neck fracture (Dyer, Ashton, & Teasdale, 1995). A prospective study found that postoperative delirium went unrecognized by physicians 80% of the time, and that nurses missed it 32% of the time (Gustafson, Brannstrom, Norberg, Bucht, & Winblad, 1991). The occurrence of postoperative delirium has been associated with the use of meperidine, epidural analgesia and anticholinergic drugs such as antiemetics (Marcantonio et al., 1994; Williams-Russo, Urquhart, Sharrock, & Charlson, 1992).

SUMMARY

The pain associated with osteoporosis may range from the dull and chronic pain associated with previous fractures and gradual vertebral disintegration to the acute excruciating pain associated with hip fractures and compression fractures of the vertebrae. Additionally, the pain may be time-limited, as in the postoperative period following surgical repair of hip fractures, or never-ending and therefore particularly draining, which is the more usual case. Because the pain is likely to increase as the osteoporotic sequelae advance over time, pain management is complicated by age-related problems associated with delay of medication metabolism and excretion. That, plus the tendency of both society and professional caregivers to discount the experience of pain in elders, place persons with osteoporosis at substantial risk for under treatment of their pain. Granted, the chronic pain associated with osteoporosis may be subtle and difficult to assess. However, failure to alleviate pain is unacceptable, and heightened attention must be given to solving this problem in all populations, but most especially in those with osteoporosis who have too long borne their pain alone.

REFERENCES

Baillie, S. P., Bateman, D. N., Coates, P. E., & Woodhouse, K. W. (1989). Age and the pharmacokinetics of morphine. *Age and Ageing, 18*, 258–262.

Benzon, H. T., Wong, H. Y., Belavic, A. M. Jr., Goodman, I., Mitchell, D., Lefheit, T., & Locicero, J. (1993). A randomized, double-blind comparison of epidural fentanyl infusion versus patient-controlled analgesia with morphine for post-thoracotomy pain. *Anesthesia and Analgesia, 76*, 316–322.

Borneman, T., & Ferrell, B. R. (1996). Ethical issues in pain management. In B. A. Ferrell (Ed.), *Clinics in geriatric medicine* (pp. 615–628). Philadelphia: W. B. Saunders.

Boulanger, A., Choiniere, M., Roy, D., Boure, B., Chartrand, D., Choquette, R., & Rousseau, P. (1993). Comparison between patient-controlled analgesia and intra-muscular meperidine after thoracotomy. *Canadian Journal of Anaesthesia, 40*, 409–415.

Brescia, F. J. (1987). A study of controlled-release oral morphine (MS Contin) in an advanced cancer hospital. *Journal of Pain and Symptom Management, 2*, 193–198.

Brown, D. L. (1985). Postoperative analgesia following thoracotomy: Danger of delayed respiratory depression. *Chest, 88*, 779–780.

Chrischilles, E. A., Lemke, J. H., Wallace, R. B., & Drube, G. A. (1990). Prevalence and characteristics of multiple analgesic use in an elderly study group. *Journal of the American Geriatrics Society, 38*, 979–984.

Cutler, R. B., Fishbain, D. A., Rosomoff, R. S., & Rosomoff, H. L. (1994). Outcomes in treatment of pain in geriatric and younger age groups. *Archives of Physical Medicine and Rehabilitation, 75*, 457–464.

Dyer, C. B., Ashton, C. M., & Teasdale, T. A. (1995). Postoperative delirium: A review of 80 primary data-collection studies. *Archives of Internal Medicine, 155*, 461–465.

Egbert, A. M. (1996). Postoperative pain management in the frail elderly. In P. Q. Vu (Series Ed.) & B. A. Ferrell (Vol. Ed.), *Clinics in geriatric medicine: Vol. 12. Pain management* (No. 3, pp. 583–599). Philadelphia: W. B. Saunders.

Egbert, M. D., Parks, L. H., Short, L. M., & Burnett, M. L. (1990). Randomized trial of postoperative patient-controlled analgesia vs. intramuscular narcotics in frail elderly men. *Archives of Internal Medicine, 150*, 1897–1903.

Ehsanullah, R. S. B., Page, M. C., Tildesley, G., & Wood, J. R. (1988). Prevention of gastroduodenal damage induced by non-steroidal anti-inflammatory drugs—controlled trial of Ranitidine. *British Medical Journal, 297*, 1017–1021.

Ferrell, B. R., & Ferrell, B. A. (1995). Pain in elderly persons. In D. B. McGuire, C. H. Yarbro, & B. R. Ferrell (Eds.), *Cancer pain management* (2nd ed., p. 273). Boston: Jones and Bartlett.

Forman, W. B. (1996). Opioid analgesic drugs in the elderly. In P. Q. Vu (Series Ed.) & B. A. Ferrell (Vol. Ed.), *Clinics in geriatric medicine: Vol. 12. Pain management* (No. 3, pp. 489–500). Philadelphia: W. B. Saunders.

Fries, J. F., Williams, C. A., Bloch, D. A., & Michel, B. A. (1991). Nonsteroidal anti-inflammatory drug-associated gastropathy: Incidence and risk factor models. *American Journal of Medicine, 91*, 213–222.

Gift, A. (1989). Visual analogue scales: Measurement of subjective phenomena. *Nursing Research, 38*, 286–288.

Grabois, M. (1988). Chronic pain evaluation and treatment. In J. Goodgold (Ed.), *Rehabilitation medicine* (pp. 663–674). St. Louis, MO: C. V. Mosby.

Gustafson, Y., Brannstrom, B., Norberg, A., Bucht, G., & Winblad, B. (1991). Underdiagnosis and poor documentation of acute confusional states in elderly hip fracture patients. *Journal of the American Geriatrics Society, 39*, 760–765.

Gustafsson, L. L., Schildt, B., & Jacobsen, K. (1982). Adverse effects of extradural and intrathecal opiates: Report of a nationwide survey in Sweden. *British Journal of Anaesthesia, 54*, 479–486.

Harkins, S. W., & Price, D. D. (1987). Assessment of pain in the elderly. In D. C. Turk & R. Melzack (Eds.), *Handbook of pain assessment*. New York: Guiford.

Hays, H., Hagen, N., Thirlwell, M., Dhaliwal, H., Babul, N., Harsanyi, Z., & Darke, A. C. (1994). Comparative clinical efficacy and safety of immediate release and controlled release hydromorphone for chronic severe cancer pain. *Cancer, 74*, 1808–1816.

Helme, R., Katz, B., Gibson, S., Bradbeer, M., Farrell, M., Neufeld, M., & Corran, T. (1996). Multidisciplinary pain clinics for older people: Do they have a role? In P. Q. Vu (Series Ed.) & B. A. Ferrell (Vol. Ed.), *Clinics in geriatric medicine: Vol. 12. Pain management* (No. 3, pp. 563–582). Philadelphia: W. B. Saunders.

Holdsworth, M., Forman, W. B., & Nystrom, K. (1994). Transdermal fentanyl disposition in elderly subjects. *Gerontology, 40*, 32–37.

Inturrisi, C. E. (1989). Management of cancer pain: Pharmacology and principles of management. *Cancer, 63*(Suppl. 11), 2308–2320.

Kapuscinski, P., Talalaj, M., Borowicz, J., Marcinowska-Suchowierska, E., &Brzozowski, R. (1996). An analgesic effect of human calcitonin in patients with primary osteoporosis. *Materia Medica Polona, 28*, 83–86.

Koo, P. J. S. (1995). Pain. In L. Y. Young & M. A. Koda-Kimble (Eds.), *Applied therapeutics: The clinical use of drugs* (6th ed., p. 7–7). Vancouver, WA: Applied Therapeutics.

Kottke, F. J., & Lehmann, J. F. (Eds.). (1990). *Krusen's handbook of physical medicine and rehabilitation*. Philadelphia: W. B. Saunders.

Lyritis, G. P., Paspati, I., Karachalios, T., Ioakimidis, D., Skarantavos, G., & Lyritis, P. G. (1997). Pain relief from nasal salmon calcitonin in osteoporotic vertebral crush fractures. A double blind, placebo-controlled clinical study. *Acta Orthopaedica Scandinavica, 275*(Suppl. October), 112–114.

Maksymowych, W. P. (1998). Managing acute osteoporotic vertebral fractures with calcitonin. *Canadian Family Physician, 44*, 2160–2166.

Marcantonio, E. R., Juarez, G., Goldman, L., Mangione, C. M., Ludwig, L. E., Lind, L., Katz, N., Cook, E. F., Orav, E. J., & Lee, T. H. (1994). The relationship of postoperative delirium with psychoactive medications. *Journal of the American Medical Association, 272*, 1518–1522.

McCaffery, M., & Beebe, A. (1989). *Pain clinical manual for nursing practice* (pp. 649–659). St. Louis, MO: C. V. Mosby.

McGuire, D. B. (1988). Measuring pain. In F. Stromborg (Ed.), *Instruments for clinical nursing research* (pp. 333–352). Norwalk, VA: Appleton and Lange.

Melzack, R. (1987). The short form McGill Pain Questionaire. *Pain, 30,* 191–197.

Miller, K. M., & Perry, P. A. (1990). Relaxation technique and postoperative pain in patients undergoing cardiac surgery. *Heart and Lung, 19,* 136–146.

Nguyen, D. M. T. (1996). The role of physical medicine and rehabilitation in pain management. In P. Q. Vu (Series Ed.) & B. A. Ferrell (Vol. Ed.), *Clinics in geriatric medicine: Vol. 12. Pain management* (No. 3, pp. 517–529). Philadelphia: W. B. Saunders.

Nyska, M., Shapira, Y., Klin, B., Drenger, B., & Margulies, J. Y. (1989). Epidural methadone for analgesic management of patients with conservatively treated proximal femoral fractures. *Journal of the American Geriatrics Society, 37,* 980–982.

Parmelee, P. A., Smith, B., & Katz, I. R. (1993). Pain complaints and cognitive status among elderly institution residents. *Journal of the American Geriatrics Society, 41,* 517–522.

Penn State Geisinger Health System Formulary Steering Committee (1999). COX-2 selective inhibitors: Celecoxib (Celebrex®) and Rofecoxib (Vioxx®). *Penn State Geisinger Health System Pharmacy and Therapeutics Review.* Danville, PA: Penn State Geisinger Health System.

Portenoy, R. F., & Farkash, A. (1988). Practical management of nonmalignant pain in the elderly. *Geriatrics, 5,* 29.

Robinson, M. G., Griffin, J. W., Bowers, J., Kogan, F. J., Kogut, D. G., Lanza, F. L., & Warner, C. W. (1989). Effect of Ranitidine gastroduodenal mucosal damage induced by nonsteroidal anti-inflammatory drugs. *Digestive Diseases & Science, 34,* 424–428.

Rowe, W. L., Goodwin, A. P., & Miller, A. J. (1992). The efficacy of pre-operative controlled-release indomethacin in the treatment of postoperative pain. *Current Medical Research and Opinion, 12,* 662–667.

Short, L. M., Burnett, M. L., Egbert, A. M., & Parks, L. H. (1990). Medicating the postoperative elderly: How do nurses make their decisions? *Journal of Gerontological Nursing, 16,* 12–17.

Silverstein, F. E., Graham, D. Y., Senior, J. R., Davies, H. W., Struthers, B. J., Bittman, R. M., & Geis, G. S. (1995). Misoprostol reduces serious gastrointestinal complications in patients with rheumatoid arthritis receiving nonsteroidal anti-inflammatory drugs: A randomized, double-blind, placebo-controlled trial. *Annals of Internal Medicine, 123,* 214–249.

Smallman, J. M., Powell, H., Ewart, M. C., & Morgan, M. (1992). Ketorolac for postoperative analgesia in elderly patients. *Anaesthesia, 47,* 149–152.

Smith, C. (1995). Upper gastrointestinal disorders. In L. Y. Young & M. A. Koda-Kimble (Eds.), *Applied therapeutics: The clinical use of drugs* (6th ed., pp. 23–13). Vancouver, WA: Applied Therapeutics.

Stahlgren, L. R., Trierweiler, M., Tommeraasen, M., Mehlisch, D., Otterson, W., Maneatis, T., Bynum, L., & DiGiorgio, E. (1993). Comparison of ketorolac and meperidine in patients with postoperative pain: Impact on health care utilization. *Clinical Therapeutics, 15*, 57–183.

Stein, W. M., & Ferrell, B. A. (1996). Pain in the nursing home. *Clinics in Geriatric Medicine, 12*, 601–613.

Walts, L. F., Kaufman, R. D., Moreland, J. R., & Weiskopf, M. (1985). Total hip arthroplasty: An investigation of factors related to postoperative urinary retention. *Clinical Orthopaedics and Related Research, 194*, 280–282.

Weller, R., Rosenblum, M., Conard, P., & Gross, J. B. (1991). Comparison of epidural and patient-controlled intravenous morphine following joint replacement surgery. *Canadian Journal of Anaesthesia, 38*, 582–586.

Williams-Russo, P., Urquhart, B. L., Sharrock, N. E., & Charlson, M. E. (1992). Postoperative delirium: Predictors and prognosis in elderly orthopedic patients. *Journal of the American Geriatrics Society, 40*, 759–767.

Woodforde, J. M., & Merskey, H. (1972a). Personality traits of patients with chronic pain. *Journal of Psychosomatic Research, 16*, 167–172.

Woodforde, J. M., & Merskey, H. (1972b). Some relationships between subjective measures of pain. *Journal of Psychosomatic Research, 16*, 173–178.

11

Adapting Clothing to Accommodate Body Changes

Janice Penrod

> I have completely come to terms with the degree of disability that I must live with. I know I'll never recover the loss of height. I'll never run or jump again. I'll always feel acutely the slightest lump in a mattress. (Bill [husband] likens me to the fabled princess who could feel a pea through several mattresses!) I'll never recover my girlish figure, and I've managed to adjust my wardrobe accordingly. In short, I can now "accentuate the positive" and be thankful for the things I can do, rather than constantly lament the things I can't.
>
> —P. Horner

Consider the changes in one's self-image that intrude as the deformity of osteoporosis advances on the body. Imagine seeing your changed body as you walk past a mirror or storefront window. Now hunched over instead of upright, the altered image changes what others see, and ultimately alters how you see your changed self.

Even the descriptive language is telling. The kyphotic curvature of the spine is referred to as a "dowager's hump." But, what is a dowager? It is

149

an elderly widow who lives off her inheritance. A picture of vitality? No. A positive image of aging? No. An image that captures the essence of the person inside? Probably not. Rather, the body, changed by the course of this disease, assumes an almost classic picture of old age. The body becomes somewhat unfamiliar, deformed. Most important, despite improvement in bone mass, this deformity will not change. It will not go away. It will change the person's life forever.

Consider: How would such a structural change affect your clothing? As the waistline expands to accommodate the organs pushed down by the lowered rib cage, pants, skirts, and dresses no longer fit around the middle. Yet the legs and buttocks have not grown into the larger sizes needed to fit the waist. The osteoporotic shift affects the torso, the trunk length shortens, making the person appear "short-waisted." The waists of standard-cut trousers now creep up toward the breastbone, or sag in the backside.

The pronounced curvature of the back creates another set of issues. As garments are pulled up and over the hump, the back of the garment shortens while the front drapes over the concave chest and appears inordinately lengthened. Form-fitting jackets or dresses take on an unbecoming look. Hemlines also highlight the structural shifts, as clothing seems to be too long in the front and too short in the back. Closures may accentuate this problem. For example, a full front zipper may buckle or heave, accentuating the postural changes. Think also of how many styles this changed body can no longer wear. You can begin to imagine the impact of these changes on the lives of people living with osteoporosis. This is not to say that there are not fashionable garments that accommodate these changes in the physical body. But for many the style of dress and ease of purchasing clothing become additional aspects of life that require accommodation. Listen to the words of a woman with osteoporosis:

> Finding clothes to conform to this structural realignment was another problem. Any close-fitting garment was now three or four inches too small around the middle and everything that was still wearable had to be shortened. It was a constant trial to have to remodel or buy clothes that would present a reasonably neat appearance. (Horner, 1989, p. 9)

This "constant trial" may not be so pressing for casual at-home wear, but what of more formal events, like a family wedding or anniversary? What of business attire that once perhaps contributed significantly to the self-image? How many of us could shift our fashion styles to accommodate these changes without some sense of loss?

Special Fashion Considerations

"You are what you wear" is an adage that has crept into our heads and captures our society's fascination with wearing apparel. Many women with osteoporosis report withdrawing from social circles, not only because of environmental concerns or physical discomfort, but also because they cannot find clothing to suit the occasion. They simply feel unpresentable, so choose not to become involved. The significance of clothing and appearance warrants special attention in considering how one may minimize the disablement of osteoporosis.

The National Osteoporosis Foundation (1998) produced a fashion guidebook for women with osteoporosis. Many of their suggestions can also be adapted for men who suffer with osteoporosis. Basically, the fashion adaptations center about five basic steps:

1. Choose silhouettes and colors that complement your style
2. Assess your current wardrobe
3. Accessorize to highlight your assets
4. Find what design elements work best for you
5. Select clothes with those elements

CHOOSE SILHOUETTES AND COLORS THAT COMPLEMENT YOUR STYLE

It is well known that certain colors and styles can hide "flaws in or out." For example, black is slimming while horizontal stripes are not. Similarly, styles that flow rather than conform to the figure can be used to disguise the postural changes of osteoporosis. A dress cut in a loosely fitting A-line that drops from the shoulders or a more flowing tent dress tend to de-emphasize the changed curvature of the spine. The shortened length of the torso may be camouflaged by a princess cut with long vertical seams, or by a tunic cut with shoulder padding and a long straight cut to the skirt. Such styles create the illusion of a longer, straighter silhouette.

Color may similarly create illusions that accentuate the positive. For example, a solid color may create a more flowing line than a garment with different colored panels. A color around the neckline will pull the eyes upward, toward the face and away from the torso. Similarly, certain colors will accentuate the eyes or hair, and will pull the eyes from nagging concerns in the silhouette. Use these colors to direct the gaze and to create the image of flow to the garment.

ASSESS YOUR CURRENT WARDROBE

Don't automatically discard the old! Much of an existing wardrobe can be altered or accessorized quite effectively. Do discard those shoes that don't provide needed support or stability. Lose the roomy purses that seem to fill with everything heavy!

Alterations may be required to retrofit clothing to the new body. Hemming can get tricky as the hemlines are often offset, front to back. Hem-marking devices may be helpful, a friend or family member may be a good assistant, or professional alterations may be in order. Most often, alterations are much less expensive than replacement, and favorite outfits can often be retained.

Another alteration technique that may come in handy is the dart. Some women call these "tucks," created as the material is folded over and sewn into place to change the contour of the garment. Darts are usually found around the tops of women's fitted garments. Now, consider using darts around the back of neckline to recontour the garment over the back. Some assistance will be needed to help pin the alterations in place, but many home seamstresses can easily manage these alterations.

Shoulder pads can also help re-form the shoulder silhouette line. Pads can be sewn into place to maximize their effect in creating a smooth line that minimizes changes to the waistline. Experiment with varied sizes of pads to create the desire look in existing garments.

ACCESSORIZE TO HIGHLIGHT YOUR ASSETS

Using scarves or jewelry, one can effectively redirect the gaze toward a glowing face or beautiful eyes. Scarves may be tied in a variety of ways to create different images. For example, a large square scarf may be folded diagonally into a triangle, draped loosely over the shoulders, and tied in front to draw the eyes upward toward the face. Scarves tied in a loose ascot can cover the changed posture of the neck area to again refocus the gaze toward the beauty of the scarf's color or design, or toward the face. Long rectangular scarves may elongate and add to the flow of the silhouette. With a little practice these techniques can serve fashion needs very well.

Jewelry can also be used to pull the gaze away from deformity. An eye-catching brooch placed near the neck or shoulder will pull the eyes toward the piece. Such jewelry need not be expensive or large and showy—just well-placed to create the image desired. Earrings may be used to frame the face and pull the eyes about the face. Watch dangling earrings that may entangle in clothing and create momentary imbalance. Long necklaces may accentuate the flow created by certain styles. Other cuts may be more suited to a shorter strand of pearls or a plain chain near the neckline. There are no rights or wrongs!

Other accessories include hats, shoes, belts, and purses. While some may use hats to frame the face, others may not be able to wear a hat because postural changes make the brim occlude vision. Fashionable footwear can be supportive and functional. Many stylish, even formal styles of footwear are available with low heels. If heels are to be worn, maximize support with a wide heel of modest height. Belts that cinch and accentuate the waistline usually do not contribute to the silhouette that these fashions attempt to create. However, a chain or cloth belt that drapes may elongate the look without accentuating the changes in the waistline. Experimentation and personal taste will help women to tailor their use of accessories to skillfully create a silhouette and pull the gaze where they want it.

Purses and handbags deserve special attention. For safety reasons, large bulky purses that must be carried by the hand or on the arm are not the best choices for women with osteoporosis. Small stylish bags that are light and can be carried with a shoulder strap can contribute to a long sleek silhouette. Backpacks or bags fashioned with dual shoulder straps that reposition the weight of the bag are often most comfortable and safest for these women. Switching handbags may be a difficult accommodation for some women, but this safety precaution may be well worth the effort.

FIND WHAT DESIGN ELEMENTS WORK BEST FOR YOU AND SELECT CLOTHES WITH THOSE ELEMENTS

Once a style that works is discovered, maximize its use. Different sleeve cuts may be preferred for comfort and appearance. For example, some may prefer a raglan cut while others prefer a wider, dropped sleeve. Different necklines may work for different body types and personal preferences. Some may prefer a tailored jeweled neckline, while others opt for a mock turtleneck or a cowl neck. The important message here is to find something that works, and then capitalize on it.

For many women, this means paying attention to details that previously were unimportant. Perhaps the best way to analyze what design elements are best is to put on an outfit that "works." Then take a good look at it. What about this outfit makes it happen? Is it color? Cut? Fabric? Accessories? Take the time to determine these elements, then use them to maximize the desired look and feel of clothing.

Above all, consider safety and comfort. Avoid skirt and trouser lengths that pose tripping hazards, shoes that don't give adequate support, or a style that looks good but feels horrid. And in regard to comfort, it is important to feel comfortable not only with the feel of the clothing, but also with the projected image. The bodies of women with osteoporosis have changed, sometimes drastically. The challenge is to use fashion to allow the inner woman to continue to shine through these unwanted physical changes.

Men Use Fashion, Too

The above guidelines have implications for men, too. Although it may seem at first glance that men are more limited than women in the range of design elements available in "on-the-rack" clothing, there is actually a rather wide variety of styles available for men. Again, it will require special attention to what works for that man. Trousers cut with a high waist will probably accentuate the trunk shortening produced by osteoporosis. Pleats may help accommodate the expanded waist while allowing the trousers to flow in a smoother silhouette.

Jackets of varied lengths are available. Longer cuts can contribute to a desirable elongated trunk silhouette. Double-breasted jackets or a three- or four-button jacket with a higher neckline may draw the eyes toward the man's face rather than to the misshaped torso. Contrasting material or color on the collar, for example a plain leather or suede collar on a patterned wool jacket, may help to frame the face and pull the gaze. Shoulder pads can help create a smoother line to the jacket. Tucks may be added to make the back of the neck fit better.

Shirts are also available in varied styles. If the standard dress shirt collar gapes or creates a bunching in the front, try a collarless shirt that does not require a tie for another look. Fitted shirts that tailor the cut to new body contours may be an option. Or, skillful tucking of excess shirt material under the arms or in the back can be used to create a smooth appearance to the shirtfront.

Accessories include standard neckties that can add color and interest to the look. Special attention may be required to knot the tie to produce a length that is neither too short nor too long. Some men may be comfortable wearing an ascot rather than a traditional necktie. As with women's fashion, the ascot can pull the gaze toward the face, toward the natural assets of the man. Lapel pins can also pull the gaze in a desired direction. Casual loose-fitting vests may camouflage changes in the trunk quite nicely.

Men also may benefit from the experience of a tailor or seamstress for altering the existing wardrobe. The same guidelines apply: look at what is available in the wardrobe, get to know what works, and maximize use of those elements through alterations or purchases. And, through it all, keep safety in mind. As the posture shifts, pants sometimes seem to take on a life of their own, growing in length. Careful attention to hemming may prevent devastating trips and falls. Dapper hats must not occlude vision, despite their contribution to a desired look.

Of greatest importance, clinicians and informal caregivers must not overlook the importance of style and fashion to their male clients. Neither osteoporosis nor fashion is an exclusively female concern. Learning the tricks of the trade will help men to maintain a self-image that promotes continued social interaction and esteem.

REFERENCES

Horner, P. (1989). *The long road back: One woman's story.* Ottawa, Canada: University of Ottawa Press.

National Osteoporosis Foundation. (1998). *Style wise: A fashion guide for women with osteoporosis.* Washington, DC: Author.

12

Target Groups for Prevention and Early Detection

Sarah Hall Gueldner

An ounce of prevention is worth a pound of cure.

—Anonymous

The evidence is overwhelming that prevention of osteoporosis is a more attainable goal than either cure or restoration. While new and developing pharmaceutical interventions are promising, none yet offers a miracle cure. Likewise, genetic-based intervention may someday be available, but it will not come quickly. What we are coming to understand is that osteoporosis is not just a part of aging that half of the world's women and 13% of its men must accept as the going price of longevity. Research findings have provided us with the knowledge needed to prevent and halt the process of bone loss in most individuals at risk.

However, prevention efforts are hampered by long-standing and deeply entrenched public and professional complacency. The first and almost daunting task is to overcome the prevailing notion that nothing can be done. We must launch a stirring informational campaign to jar the public, including the professional community, out of apathy and into focused and effective action.

This chapter addresses the process of prevention in two ways. Research findings about osteoporosis will be reviewed in order to determine the most glaring and preventable risk factors and the populations at greatest risk. Secondly, comments will be offered regarding a prevention campaign, including avenues for reaching the targeted populations.

The most prominent population at risk, overshadowing others, is that of perimenopausal women. Clearly, this population has already called some attention to itself in terms of sheer numbers. But other critical groups at risk are emerging as well. For instance, we are beginning to see that older men are at considerable risk, but their plight has so far been shamefully neglected in terms of research and treatment efforts. Likewise, the emerging and unique population of surviving and thriving transplantees have slipped up on society and may represent the most assuredly at risk group of all. Others are placed at risk by specific medical conditions such as small bowel disorders that interfere in a variety of ways with absorption of calcium, vitamin D, and other nutrients essential to bone health. The group that seems needlessly at risk, and the one we should start our prevention efforts with, are those who just do not eat enough calcium, vitamin D, and or other nutrients. A conspicuous subgroup in this category is the near epidemic number of young women who become anorexic or bulimic in search of modern society's goddess of thinness. Finally, it is perhaps in the children of the world that our best shot for prevention of osteoporosis rests. For we are finally coming to see that "osteoporosis is a childhood disease that manifests itself in older life."

Finally, the discussion related to prevention will be extended to include brief comments regarding the reduction, in as much as is possible, of the devastating consequences and sequelae, including falls and physical deformity, in those who have established osteoporosis.

Diagnostic measures of bone mass have recently become portable, allowing the potential for wide-scale screening of populations at risk. Simultaneously, major wide-scale studies like the National Osteoporosis Risk Assessment (NORA) project (1998) have begun to provide the information we need to stop this epidemic early in the new millennium. For instance, there is growing evidence that:

1. Maximizing peak bone mass in childhood and the early teen years (prepuberty) may help to prevent osteoporosis in later years.

2. Achievement of peak bone mass can be increased through attention to diet and mild impact exercise.

3. Genetic predisposition to osteoporotic bone loss is a major factor, but it need not be the seal of doom.

4. Women are at high risk for bone loss during their early postmenopausal years, but hormonal replacement therapy (HRT) and calcium with Vitamin D supplementation can slow the process of bone loss.

5. Long-term use of certain medications, such as steroids and anticonvulsants, places persons of either gender at great risk for developing osteoporosis.

6. Food sources are the best sources of absorbable calcium.

7. People of all ages should drink milk and eat other foods rich in calcium.

8. It is never too late to make a difference.

9. Some diseases, such as renal, thyroid, and gastrointestinal malabsorption disorders, increase one's risk of becoming osteoporotic.

10. Portable and relatively inexpensive diagnostic measures of bone mineral density are now available for wide-scale screening (and are now covered by most medical reimbursement plans).

11. Therapeutic pharmaceutical products are becoming available to slow, and even reverse to some degree, the silent process of osteoporotic bone destruction.

Given these increasing options, we must no longer stand by while osteoporosis robs our grandparents of their potential quality of life. Something can now be done about it at all levels. Nutritional measures and pharmaceutical products are available to prevent and/or slow the bone loss. Both public and personal environments can be modified to prevent devastating falls that end in hip fractures. We can help them find fashions that accommodate their deformed posture and preserve their self-esteem.

But, the greatest challenge to us as health professionals, and by far the most important if we are to eliminate the problem of osteoporosis in future generations, is that we design and implement a powerful global prevention campaign with the children of the world. We must teach them to choose foods high in calcium and to drink milk instead of soft drinks. We must teach to exercise regularly and not to begin smoking. Finally, we must abolish society's fetish for thinness that makes our children and young girls engage in severe dieting and anorexia. Milk is almost always replaced with calorie-free drinks in weight-reduction diets.

To their credit, the food industry has begun to produce and market calcium-enriched foods, such as orange juice, yogurt, and even water. Their efforts should be acknowledged and encouraged.

A beneficial trend in society over the past two decades is the increased participation of girls and women in competitive sports. Our still scant body of research suggests that this more active lifestyle will enhance the development of peak bone mass of girls during elementary through high school years and in college. However, it should be noted that girls who engage in very demanding training programs may develop amenorrhea leading to significantly reduced hormonal levels, which may place them at risk in terms of bone development. Likewise, it is important to remember that the girls and women who are unable or choose not to engage in competitive sports or exercise will remain at risk for developing osteoporosis. It is also important to monitor the societal impact of increased computer time on the activity levels of children and youth of both genders.

We must also strive for earlier detection. The emerging research base provides us with screening imperatives that can be implemented immediately. Fortunately, a number of the detection strategies do not depend on sophisticated technology. For instance, the simplest predictor of risk for osteoporosis, documented loss of height, requires only a ruler. As professionals, parents, and teachers we should measure the height of every citizen on the face of the earth at least once a year—without shoes on. Mothers and grade school teachers keep that information on children until somewhere around junior high school, then they may never be measured again. Whereas most of us know our weights to within a pound or two, we tend to assume we are the height that is listed on our driver's license. Accurate measurement of the height of adults is still the most ready to hand and least expensive screening procedure for osteoporosis.

Likewise, several simple pencil and paper questionnaires for assessing risk for osteoporosis are available and easy to administer, even to groups. These should be administered to the individuals sitting in every primary care waiting room and in schools, churches, and all community settings where older adults congregate.

We must make the emerging diagnostic technology available to all of the population, as we have finally done with mammography. For instance, it is not unreasonable for young women to have a portable measure of bone density when they turn 30 years of age, followed by another at the time of menopause. Those who are found to have osteopenia or osteoporosis should continue to have bone density measures thereafter as often as needed to monitor the degree of bone loss and effectiveness of therapy.

Those diagnosed with osteoporosis or osteopenia should be counseled and placed on aggressive therapeutic management programs. Additionally, fall prevention programs should be instituted, based on principles of environmental safety in both the home and public places.

If the campaign against osteoporosis is to be successful, health-related professionals must join forces with community action groups, including teachers, social agencies, media representatives, and legislators. We must infiltrate the public's eyes and ears with the message that osteoporosis is not just an unfortunate part of aging. It is taking too great a toll on our lives and resources and can be eliminated.

Primary prevention strategies are proposed for perimenopausal women, children and adolescents of both genders, elderly men, and individuals who are taking corticosteroids or anticonvulsants to treat specific medical conditions. The research based strategies for perimenopausal women are presented in other chapters and will not be repeated in this section. However, key research findings for each of the other targeted groups are summarized in this chapter. Particular attention is given to the findings related to children, adolescents, and men, since the research base for these populations has just begun to reveal data.

CHILDREN AND ADOLESCENTS

Data are just beginning to establish normal values for bone mass during childhood. These data tell us that sex differences are not seen at ages 1 through 4 but become obvious at ages 5 and 6 (Specker et al., 1987; Mazess & Cameron, 1972).

It has been shown by biochemical markers of both bone resorption (TRAP, dipyridinoline cross-links) and bone formation (bone alkaline phosphatase, osteocalcin, and the carboxyterminal propeptide of type I collagen) that bone turnover is markedly increased during childhood. These markers are present during early childhood in levels that are twice as high as in adults but decrease after puberty (Hillman, Cassidy, Johnson, Lee, & Allen, 1994).

Intestinal absorption of calcium appears to be regulated by the need for minerals for bone turnover at all ages. For instance, calcium absorption is high during infancy and adolescence, when skeletal growth is most rapid, and decreases during childhood and young adulthood (Matkovic & Heaney,

1992; Abrams & Stuff, 1994). However, research findings suggest that children from populations with chronically low calcium diets (i.e., children living in China and India) seem to be able to increase the percentage of calcium absorption (Lee, Leung, Fairweather, et al., 1994; Begum & Pereira, 1969). It is not known if this observed ability to increase calcium absorption is related to individual chronic adaptations or ethnic population differences that have evolved over generations. The data of Matkovic and Heaney (1992) show that there is a threshold effect for calcium at all ages, and that after a certain intake, balance plateaus regardless of increasing intake. These thresholds have been established at 1,090 mg for infants, 1,390 mg for children, 1,480 for adolescents, and 957 for young adults. It has also been shown that urinary calcium excretion increases with age (Matkovic & Heaney, 1992). Although muscular strength was significantly correlated with bone mass, body weight was the strongest predictor of peak bone mass (Southard et al., 1991).

Data have shown that most children meet the recommended daily requirement for calcium up to age 11 to (800 mg). However, research has shown that only 15% of girls, 11 to 24 years, meet the recommended calcium intake (1,200 mg), and that barely more than half (53%) of boys in this age category meet this standard. Regrettably, it has been shown that girls of that age take in as little as 450 mg of calcium per day (Hillman, 1996, p. 460), which is little more than half of the recommended amount.

A number of intervention trials in prepubertal children and adolescents, including a rigorously controlled study of identical twins, have demonstrated increased bone mineral density, particularly of the radius and lumbar spine, following calcium supplementation (Andon, Lloyd, & Matkovic, 1994; Chan, 1991; Johnson et al., 1992; Lee, Leung, Wang, et al., 1994; Lloyd et al., 1993; Matkovic et al., 1990). The findings approached but did not attain significance in the hip. However, these findings could not be demonstrated after puberty. It should be kept in mind that this area of research is just beginning, and follow-up studies are needed before benefits of childhood supplementation can be assumed for adult peak bone mass (Halioua & Anderson, 1989; Sandler et al., 1985).

One important study demonstrated a relationship between childhood bone density and childhood fracture rates (Chan, Hess, Hollis, & Book, 1984). Since the high fracture rate in children and adolescents has traditionally been assumed to be related to high risk behaviors in this group, it is important that more research be directed to study the effect of childhood bone mass on the incidence of childhood fractures.

Similarly, preliminary data suggest that exercise in childhood is important to the development of peak bone mass (Slemenda, Miller, Hui, Reister, & Johnston, 1991). A study involving a population of Danish youth concluded that weight bearing activity was a stronger contributor to peak bone mass than dietary intake (Welten et al., 1994). Given the potential for prevention, there is a critical need for further study in this area.

Finally, there is evidence suggesting that excess bone resorption during pregnancy may not be a characteristic of the mature woman who has achieved full maximal bone mass, but that pregnancy at an earlier age, when the skeleton of both the fetus and the mother are maturing simultaneously, may result in lower bone density and increased risk for perimenopausal bone loss (Sowers, Wallace, & Lemke, 1985; Sowers et al., 1992; Fox et al., 1993). This finding has important implications regarding both nutrition and lifestyle during adolescent years.

MEN

Overshadowed by the traditional view of osteoporosis as a disease of women, osteoporosis in men has only recently been recognized as a public health concern (Niewoehner, 1993; Scane, Sutcliffe, & Francis, 1992). It is estimated that approximately 30% of hip fractures worldwide will occur in men (Cooper, Campion, & Melton, 1992). In the U.S., the ratio of hip fractures in men over 65 years of age to women is 1:2 (Bacon, Smith, & Baker, 1989; Jacobsen et al., 1990). In southern Europe, men have as many hip fractures as women (Chalmers & Ho, 1970; Kanis, 1993); and in Singapore, the male:female ratio may even be reversed (Solomon, 1968). African-American men experience hip fractures at half the rate of Caucasians (Jacobsen et al.), and Japanese men have a lower rate of hip fracture than Caucasian men from the United States (Ross et al., 1991). Research findings show that taller, heavier men have more hip fractures, perhaps related to the force of the impact on falling (Hemenway, Azrael, Rimm, Feskanich, & Willett, 1994). It has been well-established that boys accrue bone mass for a longer period of time than girls (Bonjour, Theintz, Law, Slosman, & Rizzoli, 1994), and that all skeletal dimensions are larger in men than in women.

Once thought to be uncommon, the incidence of osteoporotic vertebral fracture in U.S. men is now believed to be at least half that of women (Mann, Oviatt, Wilson, Nelson, & Orwoll, 1992); and one study actually found the incidence to be higher in elderly men (75 years or older) than in women (O'Neill, Valow, & Cooper, 1993). Bone mineral density values are lower in men with vertebral fractures than in nonfractured men, indicating that the fractures are not caused by trauma alone (Mann et al., 1992). The occurrence of a distal forearm or tibial fracture in a man signals considerably increased risk of subsequent hip fracture, presumably due to low bone mass or increased risk of falling (Karlsson, Hasserius, & Obrant, 1993; Mallmin et al., 1993).

Studies suggest a correlation between loss of bone density in men and a decrease in gonadal function, specifically testosterone, associated with aging or treatment regimens for specific disease conditions that intentionally reduce androgen levels (Murphy, Khaw, Cassidy, & Compston, 1992: Vermculen, 1991; Vermeulen & Kaufman, 1992). More recent research findings suggest that, in addition to androgens, a deficiency in endogenous estrogens may also be of major importance for skeletal health in boys and men (Metzger & Kerrigan, 1994). Hypogonadism is present in 5% to 33% of men evaluated for vertebral fractures and osteoporosis (Jackson & Kleerekoper, 1990), and it has been shown that hip fractures in elderly men occur more often in the presence of hypogonadism (Stanley, Schmitt, Poses, & Deiss, 1991). Circumstances of hypogonadism include the now common pharmaceutical or surgical castration for conditions such as prostate cancer.

Long-term glucocorticoid treatment for medical conditions such as chronic lung disorders are also associated with low bone density. Lifestyle patterns such as smoking, excessive use of alcohol, and insufficient exercise have also been correlated with low bone mass in older men (Orwoll & Klein, 1996, p. 757).

HABITUAL ALCOHOL CONSUMPTION

The link between habitual alcohol consumption and bone loss has been well established in both men and women (Hernandez-Avila, Colditz, & Stampger, 1991; Israel, Orrego, & Holt, 1980; Slemenda et al., 1992), though the mechanisms by which alcohol induces bone disease in not clear. A study of the prevalence of reduced bone mass in individuals whose drinking habits have prompted them to seek medical help was found to be 25% to 50% (Diamond, Stiel, Lunzer, Wilkinson, & Posen, 1989).

TOBACCO USE

Tobacco use is associated with lowered bone mass and fractures in women (Krall & Dawson-Hughes, 1991) and with the prevalence of vertebral and hip fractures in men (Meyer, Tverdal, & Falch, 1993; Paganini-Hill, Chao, Ross, & Henderson, 1991; Seeman & Melton, 1983; Slemenda et al., 1992). In women, tobacco use is associated with lower weight, calcium absorption, and estrogen levels, all of which negatively influence bone mass (Orwoll & Klein, 1996, p. 763). One research team that studied twins reported a strong correlation between the number of cigarettes smoked and the rapidity of bone loss (Slemenda et al., 1992). Seeman and Melton (1983) found the risks of smoking and alcohol to be independent and multiplicative. Research is still scant on the effect of smoking in men, so it is still unknown whether smoking adversely affects androgen levels or other effectors of bone remodeling in men. Some believe that smoking may exert a direct toxic effect on bone metabolism (Orwoll & Klein, 1996, p. 763).

GASTROINTESTINAL DISORDERS

Small-bowel disorders interfere with the absorption of calcium, vitamin D, and other nutrients and are associated with bone disease. Some gastric disorders may speed nutrients in the bowel past their absorptive sites too quickly for absorption to occur. A particularly strong relationship has been established between gastrectomy and vertebral osteoporosis in both men and women (Francis, Peacock, Marshall, Horsman, & Aaron, 1989; Tovey, Godfrey, & Lewin, 1990). Large-bowel disorders are rarely associated with low bone mass, since the process of absorption is generally completed in the small intestine (Inoue et al., 1992).

EVALUATING MEN FOR OSTEOPOROSIS

The following points should be considered when evaluating men for osteoporosis:

1. History of an unexplainable low trauma fracture, especially of the vertebra or femur, or the incidental finding of vertebral deformity.
2. Men who present with glucocorticoid excess, alcoholism, or hypogonadism should be considered for bone mineral density testing.
3. Routine laboratory testing for men should include levels of serum creatinine, calcium, phosphorus, alkaline phosphatase, and liver function tests, as well as a complete blood count, to rule out the presence of medical conditions known to be associated with bone loss (Orwoll & Klein, 1996, pp. 767–768).

THERAPY

Guidelines for treating osteoporotic disorders in men are not yet available, since no guidelines have been established for use of pharmacological therapies for osteoporosis in men. However, there is a general assumption that the therapies developed for women may also be useful for treating men. Certainly, calcium and vitamin D supplementation are indicated for all older men as are appropriate lifestyle changes (e.g., cessation of smoking and excessive use of alcohol) to eliminate risk factors.

Likewise, preventive attention should be directed to exercise, nutrition, and other factors that enhance the development of peak bone mass during boyhood. Aggressive therapy should be instituted for men who receive steroid therapy for longer than three months, and androgen replacement therapy is generally thought to be useful in hypogonadal men.

Although men tend to achieve a higher mean dietary calcium intake than women, it is estimated that one-half of men ingest less than the 800 mg recommended daily allowance, and that many ingest far less (Morley, 1986; Orwoll & Klein, 1996, p. 754). This is particularly alarming, since data suggest that older men are at higher risk for increased parathyroid hormone levels (Young, Marcus, Minkoff, Kim, & Segre, 1987) and subnormal vitamin D levels (Orwoll & Meier, 1986) and may actually need more than the recommended daily calcium allowance (Morley, 1986). Findings surrounding the effects of calcium intake on hip fracture remain somewhat inconclusive but suggest a beneficial effect (Cooper, Barker, & Wickham, 1988; Looker, Harris, Madans, & Sempos, 1993; Lau, Donnan, Barker, & Cooper, 1988).

Exercise has been strongly related to a reduction in hip fracture rates in men (Paganini-Hill et al., 1991; Snow-Harter, Whalen, Myburgh, Arnaud, & Marcus, 1992; Wickham et al., 1989). As in women, body weight and mechanical force on the skeleton during exercise is also highly correlated with bone density in men (Meier, Orwoll, & Jones, 1984). Accordingly, there is growing consensus that the loss of bone density seen in older men may well be due in part to decline in physical activity and muscle strength, mimicking the effects of chronic disuse (Aniansson & Gustaffson, 1981; Larsson, Sjodin, & Karlsson, 1978).

OSTEOPOROSIS DUE TO GLUCOCORTICOID EXCESS

Glucocorticoid-induced osteoporosis occurs in both men and women, but it should be noted that exogenous glucocorticoid excess was found in a large study to be the most prominent secondary cause of spinal osteoporosis in men, accounting for 16%–18% of the cases identified (Francis et al., 1989). Perhaps because men have traditionally smoked and used alcohol more than women, steroid treatment for chronic obstructive pulmonary disease is particularly prevalent among men. The specific pathophysiology of glucocorticoid-induced osteoporosis is not yet fully understood.

An emerging and still largely unattended population at great risk for glucocorticoid-induced osteoporosis is the increasing number of transplant recipients. Studies have shown that persons who ingest prescribed glucocorticoids for as long as 3 months will lose bone density at a very rapid rate, particularly during the first 6 months of therapy. Since massive steroid therapy is a part of virtually every post-transplant treatment regime, it has been suggested that aggressive treatment be initiated even before the transplant occurs (see Table 12.1).

FALLS

Hip fractures are by far the most costly of all consequences, both in terms of public dollars and the personal threat to life and independence. For that reason, any discussion of prevention must include formalized efforts to prevent falls or better manage their negative outcomes in persons who have been diagnosed with osteoporosis. The reader is referred to chapter 9 for a detailed discussion on this topic. However, I would like to call attention to emerging research that has shown hip protectors to be very effective in the reduction of hip fractures associated with falls. In a controlled clinical trial in a nursing home population, it was found that the hip fracture rate was less than half as high in the group assigned to wear hip protectors than in the control group, even though the fall rate was similar. Additionally, it was found that virtually all of the residents in the experimental group who sustained fractures were not wearing their hip protectors at the time of their fall. Given these remarkable statistics and the modest cost of hip protectors, it would appear that hip protectors hold great promise as a cost-effective intervention for reducing the number of fractures from falls among older adults who are at risk.

Further discussion of research findings that guide the development of fall prevention strategies, nutritional management, exercise programs, and various application of pharmaceutical products are provided in related chapters.

TABLE 12.1 Osteoporosis in Men

I. Primary
  Senile
  Idiopathic
II. Secondary
  Hypogonadism
  Glucocorticoid excess
  Alcoholism
  Gastrointestinal disorders
  Hypercalciuria
  Smoking
  Anticonvulsants
  Thyrotoxicosis
  Immobilization
  Osteogenesis imperfecta
  Homocystinuria
  Systemic mastocytosis
  Neoplastic diseases
  Rheumatoid arthritis

Note: From "Osteoporosis in men: Epidemiology, pathophysiology, and clinical characterization" by E. S. Orwoll and R. F. Klein in *Osteoporosis.* Copyright ©1996 by Academic Press, reprinted by permission of the publisher.

REFERENCES

Abrams, S., & Stuff, J. (1994). Calcium metabolism in girls: Current dietary intakes lead to low rate of calcium absorption and retention during puberty. *Journal of Clinical Nutrition, 60,* 739–743.

Andon, M. B., Lloyd, T., & Matkovic, V. (1994). Supplementation trials with calcium citrate malate: Evidence in favor of increasing the calcium RDA during childhood and adolescence. *Journal of Nutrition, 124,* 1412S–1417S.

Aniansson, A., & Gustaffson, E. (1981). Physical training in elderly men with special reference to quadriceps muscle strength and morphology. *Clinical Physiology, 1,* 89–98.

Bacon, W. E., Smith, G. S., & Baker, S. P. (1989). Geographic variation in the occurrence of hip fractures among the elderly white U.S. population. *American Journal of Public Health, 79,* 1556–1558.

Baran, D. T. (1998). *Osteoporosis overview.* Paper presented at the National Osteoporosis Risk Assessment (N.O.R.A.) Symposium, Hershey, PA.

Begum, A., & Pereira, S. (1969). Calcium balance studies on children accustomed to low calcium intakes. *British Journal of Nutrition, 23,* 905–911.

Bonjour, J.-P., Theintz, G., Law, F., Slosman, D., & Rizzoli, R. (1994). Peak bone mass. *Osteoporosis International, 1,* 7–13.

Burke, M. S. (1998). *Osteoporosis: Disease, prevention and treatment.* Paper presented at the National Osteoporosis Risk Assessment (N.O.R.A.) Symposium, Hershey, PA.

Chalmers, J., & Ho, K. C. (1970). Geographical variations in senile osteoporosis: The association with physical activity. *Journal of Bone and Joint Surgery, 52B,* 667–675.

Chan, G., Hess, M., Hollis, J., & Book, L. (1984). Bone mineral status in childhood accidental fractures. *American Journal of Diseases of Children, 138,* 569–570.

Cooper, C., Barker, D. J., & Wickham, C. (1988). Physical activity, muscle strength, and calcium intake in fracture of the proximal femur in Britain. *British Medical Journal, 297,* 1443–1446.

Cooper, C., Campion, G., & Melton, L. J., III. (1992). Hip fractures in the elderly: A world-wide projection. *Osteoporosis International, 2,* 285–289.

Diamond, T., Stiel, D., Lunzer, M., Wilkinson, M., & Posen, S. (1989). Ethanol reduced bone formation and may cause osteoporosis. *American Journal of Medicine, 86,* 282–288.

Field-Munves, E. (1998). *Review of diagnostic technologies/interpreting BMD test results.* Paper presented at the National Osteoporosis Risk Assessment (N.O.R.A.) Symposium, Hershey, PA.

Fox, K. M., Magaziner, J., Sherwin, R., Scott, J. C., Plato, C. C., Nevitt, M., & Cummings, S. (1993). Reproductive correlates of bone mass in elderly women. *Journal of Bone Mineral Research, 8,* 901–908.

Francis, R. M., Peacock, M., Marshall, D. H., Horsman, A., & Aaron, J. E. (1989). Spinal osteoporosis in men. *Bone & Mineral, 5,* 347–357.

Halioua, L., & Anderson, J. (1989). Lifetime and calcium intake and physical activity habits: Independent and combined effects on the radical bone of healthy premenopausal Caucasian women. *American Journal of Clinical Nutrition, 49,* 534–541.

Hemenway, D., Azrael, D. R., Rimm, E. B., Feskanich, D., & Willett, W. C. (1994). Risk factors for wrist fracture: Effect of age, cigarettes, alcohol, body height, relative weight and handedness on the risk for distal forearm fractures in men. *American Journal of Epidemiology, 140,* 361–367.

Hernandez-Avila, M., Colditz, G. A., & Stampger, M. J. (1991). Caffeine, moderate alcohol intake and risk of fractures of the hip and forearm in middle-aged women. *American Journal of Clinical Nutrition, 54,* 157–163.

Hillman, L. (1996). Bone mineral acquisition in utero and during infancy and childhood. In R. Marcus, D. Feldman, & J. Kelsey (Eds.), *Osteoporosis* (p. 460). New York: Academic Press.

Hillman, L. S., Cassidy, J. T., Johnson, L., Lee, D., & Allen, S. (1994). Vitamin D metabolism and bone mineralization in children with juvenile rheumatoid arthritis. *Journal of Pediatrics, 124,* 910–916.

Horwith, M., & Bolognese, C. J. (1998). *Routine office practices/patient assessment*. Paper presented at the National Osteoporosis Risk Assessment (N.O.R.A.) Symposium, Hershey, PA.

Inoue, K., Shiomi, K., Higashide, S., Kan, N., Nio, Y., Tobe, T., Shigeno, C., Konishi, J., Okumura, H., Yamamuro, T., & Fukunaga, M. (1992). Metabolic bone disease following gastrectomy: Assessment by dual energy x-ray absorptiometry. *British Journal of Surgery, 79*, 321–324.

Israel, Y., Orrego, H., & Holt, S. (1980). Identification of alcohol abuse: Thoracic fractures on routine chest x-rays as indicators of alcoholism. *Alcoholism, 4*, 420–422.

Jackson, J. A., & Kleerekoper, M. (1990). Osteoporosis in men: Diagnosis, pathophysiology, and prevention. *Medicine, 69*, 137–152.

Jacobsen, S. J., Goldberg, J., Miles, T. P., Brody, J. A., Stiers, W., & Rimm, A. A. (1990). Hip fracture incidence among the old and very old: A population-based study of 745,435 cases. *American Journal of Public Health, 80*, 871–873.

Johnson, C., Miller, J., Slemenda, C., Reister, T., Hui, S., Christian, J., & Peacock, M. (1992). Calcium supplementation and increase in bone mineral density in children. *New England Journal of Medicine, 327*, 82–87.

Kanis, J. A. (1993). The incidence of hip fracture in Europe. *Osteoporosis International, 1*, S10–S15.

Karlsson, M., Hasserius, R., & Obrant, E. J. (1993). Individuals who sustain nonosteoporotic fractures continue to also sustain fragility fractures. *Calcified Tissue International, 53*, 229–231.

Krall, E. A., & Dawson-Hughes, B. (1991). Smoking and bone loss among postmenopausal women. *Journal of Bone Mineral Research, 6*, 331–338.

Larsson, L., Sjodin, B., & Karlsson, J. (1978). Histochemical and biochemical changes in human skeletal muscle with age in sedentary males, age 22–65 years. *Acta Physiologica Scandinavica, 103*, 31–39.

Lau, E., Donnan, S., Barker, D. J. P., & Cooper, C. (1988). Physical activity and calcium intake in fracture of the proximal femur in Hong Kong. *British Medical Journal, 297*, 1441–1443.

Lee, W. T. K., Leung, S. S. F., Fairweather, S. J., Leug, D. M., Tsang, H. S., Eagles, J., Qox, P., Wang, S. A., Xua, Y. C., & Zeng, W. P. (1994). True fractional calcium absorption in Chinese children measured with stable isotopes (^{42}Ca and ^{44}Ca). *British Journal of Nutrition, 72*, 883–897.

Lee, W., Leung, S., Wang, S., Wu, Y., Zeng, W., Lau, J., Oppenheimer, S., & Cheng, J. (1994). Double-blind, controlled calcium supplementation and bone mineral accretion in children accustomed to a low-calcium diet. *American Journal of Clinical Nutrition, 60*, 744–750.

Lloyd, T., Andon, M., Rollings, N., Martel, J., Landis, R., Demers, L., Eggli, D., Kieselhorst, K., & Kulin, H. (1993). Calcium supplementation and bone mineral density. *Journal of the American Medical Association, 270*, 841–844.

Looker, A. C., Harris, T. B., Madans, J. H., & Sempos, C. T. (1993). Dietary calcium and hip fracture risk: The NHANES I epidemiologic follow-up study. *Osteoporosis International, 3,* 177–184.

Mallmin, H., Ljunghall, S., Persson, I., Naessen, T., Krusemo, U. B., & Bergstrom, R. (1993). Fracture of the distal forearms as a forecaster of subsequent hip fracture: A population-based cohort study with 24 years of follow-up. *Calcified Tissue International, 52,* 269–272.

Mann, T., Oviatt, S. K., Wilson, D., Nelson, D., & Orwoll, E. S. (1992). Vertebral deformity in men. *Journal of Bone Mineral Research, 7,* 1259–1265.

Matkovic, J., & Heaney, R. (1992). Calcium balance during human growth: Evidence for threshold behavior. *American Journal of Clinical Nutrition, 55,* 992–996.

Matkovic, V., Fontana, D., Tominac, C., Goel, P., & Chestnut, C., III. (1990). Factors that influence peak bone mass formation: A study of calcium balance and the inheritance of bone mass in adolescent females. *American Journal of Clinical Nutrition, 52,* 878–888.

Mazess, R., & Cameron, J. (1972). Growth of bone in school children. Comparison of radiographic morphometry and photon absorptiometry. *Growth, 36,* 77–92.

Meier, D. E., Orwoll, E. S., & Jones, J. M. (1984). Marked disparity between trabecular and cortical bone loss with age in healthy men: Measurement by vertebral computed tomography and radial photon absorptiometry. *Annals of Internal Medicine, 101,* 605–612.

Metzger, D. L., & Kerrigan, J. R. (1994). Estrogen receptor blockade with tamoxifen diminishes growth hormone secretion in boys: Evidence for a stimulatory role of endogenous estrogens during male adolescence. *Journal of Clinical Endocrinology and Metabolism, 79,* 513–518.

Meyer, H. E., Tverdal, A., & Falch, J. A. (1993). Risk factors for hip fracture in middle-aged Norwegian women and men. *American Journal of Epidemiology, 137,* 1203–1211.

Morley, J. E. (1986). Nutritional status of the elderly. *American Journal of Medicine, 81,* 679–695.

Murphy, S., Khaw, K. T., Cassidy, A., & Compston, J. E. (1992). Sex hormones and bone mineral density in elderly men. *Bone & Mineral, 20,* 133–140.

Niewoehner, C. (1993). Osteoporosis in men: Is it more common than we think? *Postgraduate Medicine, 93,* 59–58.

O'Neill, T. W., Valow, J., & Cooper, C. (1993). Differences in vertebral deformity indices between 3 European populations. *Journal of Bone Mineral Research, 8,* S149.

Orwoll, E. S., & Klein, R. F. (1996). Osteoporosis in men: Epidemiology, pathophysiology, and clinical characterization. In R. Marcus, D. Feldman, & J. Kelsey (Eds.), *Osteoporosis* (pp. 745–784). San Diego, CA: Academic Press.

Orwoll, E. S., & Meier, D. E. (1986). Alterations in calcium, vitamin D, and parathyroid hormone physiology in normal men with aging: Relationship to the development of senile osteopenia. *Journal of Clinical Endocrinology and Metabolism, 63,* 1262–1269.

Paganini-Hill, A., Chao, A., Ross, R. K., & Henderson, B. E. (1991). Exercise and other factors in the prevention of hip fracture: The Leisure World study. *Epidemiology, 2,* 16–25.

Ross, P. D., Norimatsu, H., Davis, J. W., Yano, K., Wasnich, R. D., Fujiwara, S., Hosoda, Y., & Melton, L. J., III. (1991). A comparison of hip fracture incidence among native Japanese, Japanese Americans, and American Caucasians. *American Journal of Epidemiology, 133,* 801–809.

Sandler, R., Slemenda, C., LaPorte, R., Cauley, J. A., Schramm, M. M., Barresi, M. L., & Kristen, A. M. (1985). Postmenopausal bone density and milk consumption in childhood and adolescence. *American Journal of Clinical Nutrition, 42,* 270–274.

Scane, A. C., Sutcliffe, A. M., & Francis, R. M. (1992). Osteoporosis in men. *Clinical Rheumatology 7,* 589–601.

Seeman, E., & Melton, L. I., III. (1983). Risk factors for spinal osteoporosis in men. *American Journal of Medicine, 75,* 977–983.

Slemenda, C. W., Christian, J. C., Reed, T., Reister, T. K., Williams, C. J., & Johnston, C. C. J. (1992). Long-term bone loss in men: Effects of genetic and environmental factors. *Annals of Internal Medicine, 117,* 286–291.

Slemenda, G., Miller, J., Hui, S., Reister, T., & Johnston, C. (1991). Role of physical activity in the development of skeletal mass in children. *Journal of Bone Mineral Research, 6,* 1227–1233.

Snow-Harter, C., Whalen, R., Myburgh, K., Arnaud, S., & Marcus, R. (1992). Bone mineral density, muscle strength, and recreational exercise in men. *Journal of Bone Mineral Research, 7,* 1291–1296.

Solomon, L. (1968). Osteoporosis and fracture of the femoral neck in the South African Bantu. *Journal of Bone and Joint Surgery, 50B,* 2–13.

Southard, R., Morris, J., Mahan, J., Hayes, J., Torch, M., Sommer, A., & Zipf, W. (1991). Bone mass in healthy children measurement with quantitative DXA. *Radiology, 179,* 735.

Sowers, M. F. R., Clark, M. K., Hollis, B., Wallace, R. B., & Jannausch, M. (1992). Radial bone mineral density in pre- and perimenopausal women: A prospective study of rates and risk factors for loss. *Journal of Bone Mineral Research, 7,* 647–657.

Sowers, M. F. R., Wallace, R. B., & Lemke, J. H. (1985). Correlates of mid-radius bone density among premenopausal women: A community study. *Preventive Medicine, 14,* 585–596.

Stanley, H. L., Schmitt, B. P., Poses, R. M., & Deiss, W. P. (1991). Does hypogonadism contribute to the occurrence of a minimal trauma hip fracture in elderly men? *Journal of the American Geriatrics Society, 39,* 766–771.

Tovey, F. I., Godfrey, J. E., & Lewin, M. R. (1990). A gastrectomy population: 25–30 years on. *Postgraduate Medical Journal, 66,* 450–456.

Vermeulen, A. (1991). Androgens in the aging male. *Journal of Clinical Endocrinology and Metabolism, 73,* 221–223.

Vermeulen, A., & Kaufman, J. M. (1992). Editorial: Role of the hypothalamo-pituitary function in the hypoandrogenism of healthy aging. *Journal of Clinical Endocrinology and Metabolism, 75,* 704–706.

Welten, D., Kemper, H., Post, G., Van Mechelen, W., Twisk, J., Lips, P., & Teule, G. (1994). Weight-bearing activity during youth is a more important factor for peak bone mass than calcium intake. *Journal of Bone Mineral Research, 9,* 1089–1096.

Wickham, C. A. C., Walsh, K., Cooper, C., Barker, D. J. P., Margetts, B. M., Morris, J., & Bruce, S. A. (1989). Dietary calcium, physical activity, and risk of hip fracture: A prospective study. *British Medical Journal, 299,* 889–892.

Young, G., Marcus, R., Minkoff, J. R., Kim, L. Y., & Segre, G. V. (1987). Age-related rise in parathyroid hormone in man: The use of intact and midmolecule antisera to distinguish hormone secretion from retention. *Journal of Bone Mineral Research, 2,* 367–374.

13

Osteoporosis: Clinical Implications Across Disciplines

Delores C. Schoen

The prevention of osteoporosis is an attainable goal.

—D. C. Schoen

Osteoporosis is defined as "a systemic skeletal disease characterized by low bone mass and microarchitectural deterioration of bone tissue, leading to enhanced bone fragility and an increase in fracture risk" (Consensus Development Conference Report, 1993). With few exceptions, it is a systemic disorder that affects the individual's entire skeletal system. With microarchitectural deterioration, there is thinning of the bone cortex and a disappearance of the trabeculae, the supporting structures within the bone. As the trabeculae deteriorate, the bone is weakened and becomes susceptible to fracture. The skeleton may become so fragile that fractures can occur in instances where healthy bone would not break, such as bending over to pick up a newspaper, carrying a bag of groceries, turning over in bed, or even coughing or sneezing.

The prevention, detection, and treatment of osteoporosis are all areas of concern. Prevention efforts are needed for all age groups, as only 15%–20%

175

of women at high risk for osteoporosis are receiving preventive treatment. This chapter presents a brief discussion of the clinical problem, the pathology, the risk factors, the detection, the treatment, and the changing focus of prevention within different age groups.

THE PROBLEM

Osteoporosis represents a major public health problem for 28 million Americans, 80% of whom are women. In the United States today, 10 million individuals have osteoporosis, whereas 18 million more have low bone mass, placing them at increased risk for the disease. Although many people view osteoporosis as a disease of the elderly, it is important to remember that it can occur at earlier ages, and that it really begins during the years of skeletal system development. Another way of putting it is that osteoporosis is a pediatric problem that manifests itself in geriatrics.

Osteoporosis and its complications are associated with significant morbidity and mortality. It is responsible for 1.5 million fractures annually, including more than 300,000 hip, 700,000 vertebral, and 200,000 wrist fractures. As has been noted, a White woman's risk of a hip fracture is equal to her combined risk of breast, uterine, and ovarian cancer.

Today, hip fractures remain one of the most potentially devastating injuries of the elderly. The incidence of hip fracture increases with age, doubling with each decade beyond age 50, and occurring twice as often in women as in men. There is a two to three times higher incidence of hip fractures in White females than in Black and Hispanic women. A study by Lindsey and Cosman (1992) found that approximately half of the individuals who break a hip will never walk again independently, and a third will require placement in a long-term care institution. Studies by Magaziner, Simonsick, Kashner, Hebel, and Kenzora (1989) and Cummings, Black, and Nevitt (1993) found that hip fractures also result in 12%–20% mortality within the first year. The estimated national direct medical expenditures (for hospitals and nursing homes) for osteoporosis and related fractures is $13.8 billion ($38 million each day) and the cost is rising.

Despite its prevalence, severity, and cost, osteoporosis did not emerge as a major health concern until recent years. It was not until 1986 that the National Osteoporosis Foundation (NOF) was established. NOF is the only scientific and medically based nonprofit voluntary health organization dedicated to the prevention, diagnosis, and treatment of osteoporosis.

THE PATHOLOGY

Let us review the nature of the condition. Osteoporosis can be classified into two major types, primary and secondary. Primary osteoporosis is further subdivided into postmenopausal (Type I) and senile osteoporosis (Type II), with a significant overlap between the two. Secondary osteoporosis is not related to normal aging or hormone loss, but is typically caused by medication or illness. Secondary osteoporosis is present in about 20% of women and 40% of men at the time they are diagnosed with osteoporosis. A list of some of the more prevalent causes of secondary osteoporosis include endocrine problems, marrow disorders, gastrointestinal problems, collagen and genetic disorders, and specific medications, including chemotherapy, glucocorticoids, and anticonvulsants.

Patients with primary Type I osteoporosis are typically females who have lost predominately trabecular bone. The hypothesized pathogenesis is estrogen deficiency leading to an increased bone remodeling rate, increased resorption, and trabecular bone loss with frequent trabecular perforation. The increase in bone loss leads to increased plasma calcium, which suppresses parathyroid hormone secretion. Circulating vitamin D is decreased, further decreasing calcium absorption. This leads to additional bone loss as the disease progresses.

The skeleton is made up of two types of bone; 80% of it is dense cortical bone and about 20% is the spongy, trabecular bone. Individuals with Type II osteoporosis are older than those with Type I and have a roughly equal loss of cortical and trabecular bone. The hypothesized pathogenesis is an age-related decrease in hydroxylation of vitamin D by the kidney, leading to a decreased level of circulating vitamin D. This causes decreased calcium absorption by the gut which in turn stimulates a secondary hyperparathyroidism and increased bone remodeling. With the parathyroid hormone stimulated, there is increased osteoclasis and osteoblast senescence, and more bone loss results.

THE RISK FACTORS

A number of risk factors for osteoporosis have been identified. The following is only a brief review of the major ones.

Gender

Although osteoporosis affects both sexes, women are more likely to develop the disease, primarily as the result of the accelerated bone loss which occurs in women after menopause. In addition, women tend to have less bone mass than men to begin with and, therefore, less bone to lose before the fracture threshold is reached.

The peak bone mass concept needs to be reviewed. Peak bone mass refers to the maximum amount of bone a person will develop, usually by age 30. (Peak bone mass is different from maximal bone length, which occurs at approximately age 20 to 22 in males and 18 to 20 in females.) Peak bone mass is determined by a number of influences. Genetic influences (from multiple genes) determine 75%–80% of the variability, and vitamin D receptor gene polymorphism appears to have a significant effect. In general, peak bone mass is greater in men than in women and greater in Blacks than in Whites. There is a higher concordance of peak bone mass in monozygotic as opposed to dizygotic twins.

Race/Ethnicity

Non-Hispanic White and Asian individuals tend to have less bone mass and a higher risk of osteoporosis than African Americans or Hispanics. Racial and ethnic differences are just beginning to be appreciated, and there appears to be significant geographical differences in European populations.

A recent research study of both men and women across 16 European countries by Lunt et al. (1997) found that there was a clear difference in bone density and fracture risk at three anatomical sites (spine, trochanter, and femoral neck). These differences were evident between centers using the same brand of densitometer, and body size only accounted for a small fraction of the differences. For the female femoral neck data, the mean difference in the Lunt et al. (1997) study between Oviedo, Spain (the lowest site), and Harrow, England (the highest site), suggests a difference in future hip fracture risk of 2.5 to 3.0 fold. The authors suggest that these findings are the result of interactions between genetic and environmental factors. This is the first study which has shown substantial differences in bone mineral density (BMD) between different Caucasian populations after adjusting for body size.

Body Type/Genetic Factors

Slender individuals have a higher risk of osteoporosis. Several reasons seem to be involved. People with thinner, smaller bones have less bone mass to lose. Having less body weight and muscle mass results in less stress on/ stimulation of the skeleton, hence lower bone mass. Women who have less body fat also tend to produce less estrogen. Women of reproductive age whose postmenopausal mothers have osteoporosis exhibit a lower bone mineral density than women in the general population.

Exercise

Weight-bearing activity (such as walking or lifting heavy objects) tends to increase bone formation, while immobilization causes rapid bone loss. Research has shown that weight bearing and exercise increase lumbar spine bone density. In general, a regular program of exercise that includes a one-mile walk (20 to 30 minutes) three times a week will maintain bone mass. Although exercise is essential to maintain bone mass, too much exercise can have a negative impact. If young women exercise to the point that they stop menstruating, they will lose bone mass.

Nutritional Factors

There is a large body of evidence indicating that nutrition plays an important role in bone development and age-related bone loss. Calcium is the most significant factor. Inadequate dietary calcium in childhood and adolescence can prevent individuals from developing a high peak bone mass around age 30, and inadequate calcium intake in adulthood can interfere with bone rebuilding and increase bone loss. Calcium deficits at any age can result in an increased risk of osteoporosis. Besides calcium and vitamin D, the other nutrients that affect bone health include phosphorus, magnesium, and protein. High protein and high sodium diets increase urinary loss of calcium.

The usual dietary intake of calcium in the United States (450–550 mg) falls well below the adult Recommended Dietary Allowance of 1,000 to 1,500 mg per day. The calcium requirement for different ages are (a) 800–1,000 mg of calcium for ages 1 to 10, (b) 1,200 mg for ages 11 to 25, (c) 1,000 mg for ages 26 to 49, and (d) 1,500 mg for those over age 50.

Inadequate vitamin D can also interfere with bone formation. Recently the National Academy of Sciences' Institute of Medicine issued vitamin D guidelines for various age groups. They are (a) 200 iu for ages 9 to 50 years with limited sun exposure, (b) 400 iu for ages 51 to 70 with limited sun exposure, and (c) 600 iu for individuals over age 70 with limited sun exposure. Elderly patients tend to absorb calcium less efficiently, and thus 800 iu may be required.

A high-protein diet may also increase an individual's risk of developing osteoporosis. When animal protein is broken down in the body it produces acid. This acid is then buffered in the bone by releasing calcium, which is then lost through urinary excretion. It is not presently known how high the protein content of a diet must be, or for how long, to result in bone mass loss. It is also important to note that a vegetarian diet, using nonanimal protein, may actually protect against bone loss. A study by Marsh, Sanchez, Michelsen, Keiser, and Mayor (1980) compared older White women who ate meat regularly to lacto-ovo-vegetarians who ate cheese and dairy products. Those who ate the vegetarian diet lost significantly less bone with age. Both groups had a good amount of calcium in their diets, yet the meat eaters lost about a third of their bone mass between the ages of 50 and 90, while the vegetarians lost only a fourth. Another study of both men and women (Barzel, 1995) showed that vegetarians had more bone mass in their 70s than meat eaters had in their 50s. Although the reasons for the differences are not clear, a couple of hypotheses are (a) red meat is high in phosphorus and may change the phosphorus-to-calcium ratio, resulting in calcium loss, and (b) the acid levels of the two diets differ. The vegetarian diet is low in acid, while a meat diet is high. The acid has to be neutralized, and this neutralization occurs in the bone. However, a balanced diet with 45 grams of protein daily does not cause calcium loss if the ratio is maintained (i.e., 45 grams of protein plus 1,000 milligrams of calcium).

Tobacco and Alcohol Use

Chronic use of these two substances can increase the risk of osteoporosis. Both tobacco and alcohol are believed to have a toxic effect on bone or on the cells that make bone, and both have been linked with low bone mass and a higher risk of fractures. Studies have shown that smoking increases bone loss in both sexes and is known to reduce estrogen levels in women. Alcohol is a direct inhibitor of osteoblasts and may also inhibit calcium absorption.

Caffeine Use

The caffeine in tea, coffee, and soda has been linked to low bone density and higher risk of fracture in several studies. However, a recent study suggests that adequate dietary calcium may help to counterbalance the negative effects of caffeine on bone. Therefore, further study is needed to clarify a possible direct effect of caffeine on bone density. However the widespread selection of low-calorie caffeinated beverages over milk may well exert a substantial indirect effect on an individual's risk for osteoporosis.

Hormonal Factors

Estrogens help to regulate the bone remodeling process in women, and an estrogen deficiency at any age can result in increased bone loss. Women who may be at increased risk for osteoporosis because of estrogen deficiency include athletes who have stopped having menstrual periods because of strenuous training, women who have had their ovaries surgically removed, and postmenopausal women who do not use estrogen supplements.

THE DETECTION

Now that we have identified the major risk factors, we need a way to identify those with low bone mass or osteoporosis. The measurement of low bone mass encounters a number of practical problems. Early laboratory studies of blood and urine are usually within normal limits, and only after there has been a 30% loss of bone is the loss visible on x-rays.

The bone mineral density (BMD) test plays a central role in the diagnosis of osteoporosis. The BMD test is a noninvasive and accurate measurement of bone mineral density based on the fact that mineralized bone absorbs x-rays at different rates than soft tissue. Combined with population level data on bone density, the test provides two standardized scores: T and Z. The T-score is the patient's score in standard units based on values from a young adult population. The Z-score is the patient's score in standard units based on a population of the same age and sex as the patient.

The World Health Organization (WHO) defines osteoporosis in terms of bone mineral density. Normal bone density is a T-score between +1 and −1 standard deviation. Osteopenia is defined as a T-score between −1 and −2.5. Osteoporosis is considered present when the T-score is below (i.e., more negative than) −2.5. It is considered severe if the patient has had a fracture. However, the WHO distributions are based on a population of Caucasian women, and are not necessarily applicable to all groups.

There are a number of machines now available to assess bone mineral density. Quantitative computed tomography (QCT) scanning to assess vertebral BMD has an accuracy of 3%–5% in measuring bone loss. However, QCT is costly and delivers a considerable amount of radiation. The current "gold standard" for BMD testing is dual energy x-ray absorptiometry (DEXA), used in testing the hip and spine. It is precise, reasonably economical, and increasingly available. The quantitative ultrasound (QUS) is another technique that offers a low cost, ultra fast, portable, and radiation-free method for assessing bone density, especially of the os calcis, wrist, and hand.

Nonetheless, bone mineral density tests are still fairly expensive and time consuming, and some involve exposure to radiation. Most people being tested have already had fractures or have shown signs of advanced bone loss. A cheaper and more effective way to determine risk, and the need for a BMD, is a pencil and paper risk assessment tool.

Presently, the most used osteoporosis evaluation tool is the Simple Calculated Osteoporosis Risk Estimation (SCORE) tool developed by Merck and Company. SCORE has only six questions and can be administered quickly and cheaply. The tool was developed by a fairly sophisticated process. A questionnaire of approximately 60 items was developed incorporating potential risk factors identified from an extensive review of the medical literature. In the developmental stage, 1,424 peri- and postmenopausal women were asked to complete the questionnaire. Their BMD was measured by DEXA, and multivariate regression analyses were performed to determine the relationship of those risk variables to their bone mass. The six item SCORE questionnaire for postmenopausal women was then developed using the predictive factors identified by the regression model. That questionnaire was tested in a validation cohort of 208 postmenopausal women. The validation study showed that SCORE achieved 91% sensitivity (i.e., it correctly identified 91% of persons with low bone mass) and 40% specificity (i.e., it correctly classified 40% of women who did not have low bone mass).

Merck is to be commended for their work in developing the SCORE assessment tool. Still, there are a number of problems with that tool. It is only appropriate for testing postmenopausal women; it is not suitable for either younger females or for men. The assessment is limited to only six questions that deal with age, race, rheumatoid arthritis, fracture history after age 45, hormone replacement therapy, and weight. It ignores a number of other risk factors that are known to be significant, at least at the younger ages. Work still needs to be done in this area.

THE TREATMENT

The treatment plan for individuals with low bone mass focuses on exercise, calcium, vitamin D, and hormone replacement. There still remains controversy about hormone replacement because of the risk of cancer. That risk needs to be discussed with one's health care provider on a one-to-one basis. In addition, bisophosphonates (e.g., Alendrante [Fosamax]) have been utilized for low bone mass and osteoporosis treatment. Bisophosphonates slow the remodeling rate of bone and decrease resorption at each site of bone turnover. An in-depth discussion of treatment methods can be found in chapter 8.

THE PREVENTION

The prevention of osteoporosis involves maximizing peak bone density and minimizing loss of bone after peak bone mass has been reached. Major preventive measures include (a) assuring that adequate calcium and vitamin D intake is maintained throughout the life cycle, (b) engaging in weight-bearing physical activity as a lifetime endeavor, and (c) hormone replacement therapy, as appropriate, for women in the older years. For older adults with low bone density, fall prevention is an essential safety measure (see chapter 9).

THE EDUCATION OF HEALTH CARE CONSUMERS

Since osteoporosis prevention is a life-long endeavor, education efforts are needed at all ages. The following discussion presents educational strategies appropriate for different age groups, from preschool through old age.

Preschool Children (0 to 4 Years)

The education of parents has been identified as an effective way of preventing osteoporosis. Educate parents about how bones develop and remodel over the child's lifetime and the importance of developing a good peak bone mass. Eating habits established during childhood usually determine life-long dietary patterns. Many parents are not aware of their children's daily calcium requirements (birth–0.5 year—360 mg, 0.5–1 year—540 mg, and 1–10 years—800 to 1,000 mg per day) and thus may unknowingly promote eating patterns that contain inadequate calcium for optimal skeletal and bone mass development. Remember milk is not the only way to gain calcium through food. Encourage children to eat a well-balanced diet that includes green leafy vegetables, fish, and cheese (see chapter 4). Children should receive adequate vitamin D (through food and sunlight) and participate in play activities that provide weight-bearing and stress exercises appropriate for their age. Others who provide care for children, such as family members, nannies, babysitters, and day care providers, also play an important role in ensuring that these needs are met and need to be targeted for education.

It is important to inform mothers of young children, many of whom are still in their own bone development phase, about the need to increase their own peak bone mass. Young parents who are informed about osteoporosis are in a position to encourage their own mothers to implement preventive measures (and treatment as appropriate) around the time of menopause.

Encourage hospitals and clinics to include nutrition education for parents in prenatal programs. Parents, especially mothers, may be most receptive to nutrition information during their first pregnancy and should be specifically targeted for osteoporosis prevention education at that time. The education of grandparents about childhood nutritional and exercise needs can be done through the parents, as well as through the sources described under "Older Adults."

Provide education for professional child care providers on the nutrition (for meals and snacks) and exercise needs of children, appropriate for age. These should contain simple messages appropriate for both staff and parents and should include a recommendation that parents ask their children's health care providers about nutritional and exercise needs. Encourage center staff to distribute the materials to parents and to become actively involved in educating parents.

School Age Children (5 to 11 Years)

Once children have reached school age, schools become an important avenue for imparting information and helping to shape healthy behaviors regarding nutrition and exercise. The primary prevention objectives for this age group are to increase calcium intake (800 to 1,200 mg per day) and promote physical activity that involves weight bearing and stress to the muscles and skeletal system. Childhood malnutrition, which affects protein intake and prolonged vitamin D deficiency, has a significant effect on skeletal development and peak bone mass. In young females, malnutrition and poor diet delay puberty, and delayed puberty has been identified as a clear risk factor for osteoporosis.

Educational endeavors should include parents, scout leaders, teachers, administrators, food service staff, and policy makers. Suggested educational topics to include are (a) the health impact of physical activity and nutrition on bone development and disease, especially that inadequate weight-bearing activity and calcium intake can cause deficits in skeletal and bone mass development; (b) the inadequacy of current activity patterns in children for good skeletal and bone mass development; (c) the failure of current dietary patterns in children to provide adequate levels of calcium for optimal bone development; (d) the possible effects of large amounts of caffeine drinks on bone development; (e) the importance of education, nutrition, and weight-bearing exercises during the early years, since osteoporosis is a pediatric problem that manifests itself in geriatrics; (f) the relative importance of prevention for girls, who have a higher risk than boys of developing osteoporosis in their later years because they tend to have lower calcium intake and lower physical activity levels than boys; (g) the consequences of osteoporosis, including costs to society and to individuals; and (h) stress to children that milk and exercise are important for healthy bone development.

Encourage the inclusion of physical activity programs and nutritional education (that includes a discussion of daily requirements for calcium and vitamin D and how they relate to skeletal and bone mass development) in all primary and secondary school curricula. Promote educational programs related to bone mass development and the prevention of osteoporosis through youth organizations (e.g., scouts), athletic organizations, and service clubs. Provide teachers information on bone development and osteoporosis prevention through their professional organizations, publications and conferences, and parent-teacher organizations.

Adolescent Children (12 to 18 Years)

Include the educational endeavors discussed under School Age Children but also include the following: (a) dieting by eliminating milk products is a significant problem among teenage girls; (b) boys who go on very restrictive diets to maintain weight limits to participate in certain sports (i.e., wrestling and gymnastics) put themselves at risk of lower peak bone mass at age 30; (c) the possible negative effects of using a high animal protein diet to help control weight; (d) anorexia nervosa, developed by some individuals who severely restrict their diet because they fear that food will make them appear unattractive, may lead to low peak bone mass, which increases their risk of fractures throughout their lives and osteoporosis during their older years; (e) excessive training/exercise may diminish estrogen production and bone health in female athletes; (f) taking steroids for the development of muscle mass may negatively impact skeletal and bone mass development; and (g) use of alcohol and tobacco hinders bone mass development.

Points that need to be stressed to adolescent girls are (a) milk is associated with healthy, active, attractive people; (b) nonfat and low-fat dairy foods are low in calories and extremely good for your health; (c) there are nondairy foods that have high calcium content; and (d) inadequate calcium intake or physical activity can weaken bones and lead to unattractive postural deformities or hip fractures later in life.

In addition to the promotional ideas discussed previously, help inform physical education teachers and coaches, through their professional organizations, about the effects of excessive exercise on estrogen development and bone development in young female athletes. Investigate ways to use popular magazines read by adolescents to channel information regarding nutrition, exercise, estrogen, and osteoporosis to this age group. Use focus groups and promotional programs to increase high-calcium food choices by students.

Young Adults (19 to 34 Years)

Young females, because of their higher risk of developing low bone mass and osteoporosis, need to be a primary target of educational efforts. However, don't forget that the education of men is also important as a significant number of elderly men also develop osteoporosis. In addition, men need to be informed about osteoporosis so that they will support women's efforts to make changes in their lifestyle. Emphasis should be placed on increasing bone strength through nutrition and exercise, to achieve the highest possible level of bone mass by age 30. Young adults should also be targeted for education about the nutritional and activity needs of young children. Discussions should also focus on medical conditions and surgical procedures that place individuals at risk for osteoporosis and measures that can be taken to help prevent the development of secondary osteoporosis. Reinforce the need to limit the number of caffeine drinks per day, restrict the use of alcohol, and avoid tobacco.

Adults (35 to 65 Years)

In addition to the points of discussion under young adults, women over age 40 should receive information about the effects of menopause on bone mass and the need to maintain their nutritional and activity levels. They should also be aware of the rapid decrease in bone mass that occurs during the first five years after menopause. Discuss the possibility of hormone replacement therapy. Women who do not seek medical care on a regular basis need to be informed through other sources. This information may be disseminated through popular women's magazines or newsletters and journals provided through their work-related or professional organizations. Disseminate information through health and exercise clubs.

Reinforce that (a) osteoporosis can be prevented or its severity reduced through a well-balanced diet, adequate calcium intake (1000 mg per day), adequate vitamin D, participation in weight-bearing exercises, and hormone replacement; (b) most adult diets do not contain enough calcium, so calcium supplements need to be taken; (c) women are at higher risk than men; (d) non-Hispanic Caucasians and Asians are at higher risk than African Americans and Hispanics; (e) individuals who develop osteoporosis often suffer deformity, pain, and hip fractures; (f) hip fractures in older adults are usually life-changing events which can lead to restriction of activity, inability to live independently, or even death; and (g) the risk of hip fracture for women is about the same as the risk of breast, uterine, and ovarian cancer combined; hip fracture risk for men is about the same as the risk of prostate cancer.

Provide information to occupational health nurses through their professional organizations to encourage education programs and information at adult worksites. Include information about osteoporosis prevention in wellness programs. Promote the development of educational lunch time seminars at worksites to discuss the ramifications of osteoporosis. Provide prevention, detection, and treatment information about osteoporosis through (a) health fairs; (b) public service announcements on television, on radio, and in print media; (c) community service presentations through hospitals, clinics, public health agencies, health coalitions, church groups, and other organizations;

(d) educational displays at grocery stores; and (e) community seminars, possibly sponsored by pharmaceutical companies.

Older Adults (Over 65 Years)

In addition to the points addressed in the previous discussion for adults, stress the importance of calcium, physical activity, and estrogen use for adults over age 65. The prevention of falls is an increasingly important area of concern for older individuals (see chapter 9). In later years, when bone mass may be lower and balance may be more of a problem, educational messages need to emphasize the prevention of falls to reduce hip fractures from osteoporosis.

Messages to older adults need to focus on: (a) osteoporosis is more prevalent among older adults than many other diseases; (b) steps can be taken to prevent fractures no matter how much bone mass has already been lost; (c) a calcium-rich diet and vitamin D are especially important in later years because calcium absorption decreases with age; (d) it is never too late to start hormone replacement therapy; (e) physical activity is important for maintaining bone strength and provides other health benefits as well; (f) walking (20 to 30 minutes 3 times a week) is a good form of bone-strengthening exercise for most people; (g) small increases in bone mass can result in large reductions in fracture risks; (h) weight/strength training can strengthen bones, may reduce the risk of falling by improving balance, and can be done in the home using soup cans and other simple devices; and (i) some medications, poor sensory and vision problems, and environmental factors (i.e., loose rugs, items left on the floor, and poor lighting) can greatly increase an individual's risk of falling.

Provide older adults with information about available group exercise programs, such as YMCA, recreation, and senior center programs. Provide educational materials through health care provider waiting rooms, senior centers, women's groups, church groups, clubs and social organizations, congregate meal sites (especially in rural areas), senior housing facilities, and retirement groups. Provide information for publication through existing newsletters/magazines (e.g., AARP Newsletter and Prevention Magazine).

THE EDUCATION OF HEALTH CARE PROVIDERS

All health educators and care providers are in a position to help educate health care consumers regarding osteoporosis. They can influence the health behavior of individuals, both directly and indirectly, through the involvement of their professional organizations, their influence on health policy development locally and elsewhere, and their participation in educational activities at their worksite. Providers need to be updated on recent developments in osteoporosis prevention, detection, and treatment, since they have a unique opportunity to identify risk factors and provide education about prevention and treatment.

All health care providers have a role in helping other health care providers become knowledgeable and keep up-to-date on osteoporosis. Besides physicians and nurses, dietitians have a role in providing up-to-date information on nutritional (especially calcium, protein, and vitamin D) needs across the life span. Physical and occupational therapists and exercise physiologists need to provide information on weight-bearing exercises important for developing peak bone mass and preventing falls for persons of all ages. Psychologists need to provide information and strategies helpful to effect behavior change in different age groups. Health care researchers can provide cost/ benefit data on screening and treatment methods, and the care of individuals who fracture (i.e., hip, vertebra, and wrist). The prevention of osteoporosis is an attainable goal.

REFERENCES

Barzel, U. S. (1995). The skeleton as an anion exchange system: Implications for role of acid-base imbalance and genesis of osteoporosis. *Journal of Bone and Mineral Research, 10,* 1431–1436.

Conference Report. (1993). Consensus development conference: Diagnosis, prophylaxis and treatment of osteoporosis. *American Journal of Medicine, 94,* 646–650.

Cummings, S. R., Black, D. M., & Nevitt, M. C. (1993). Bone density at various sites and prediction of hip fracture in women. *Lancet, 341,* 72–75.

Lindsey, R., & Cosman, F. (1992). Primary osteoporosis. In F. Coe & M. Favus (Eds.), *Disorders of bone and mineral metabolism* (pp. 831–888). New York: Raven Press.

Lunt, M., Felsenberg, D., Adams, J., Benevolenskaya, L., Cannata, J., Dequeker, J., Dodenhof, C., Falch, J. A., Johnell, O., Khaw, K.-T., Masryk, P., Pols, H., Poor, G., Reid, D., Scheidt-Nave, C., Weber, K., Gilman, A. J., & Reeve, J. (1997). Population-based geographic variations in DXA bone density in Europe: The EVOS study. *Osteoporosis International, 7,* 175–189.

Magaziner, J., Simonsick, E., Kashner, T., Hebel, J., & Kenzora, J. (1989). Survival experience of aged hip fracture patients. *American Journal of Public Health, 79,* 274–278.

Marsh, A. G., Sanchez, T. V., Michelsen, O., Keiser, J., & Mayor, G. (1980). Cortical bone density of adult lacto-ovo-vegetarian and omnivorous women. *Journal of the American Dietetic Association, 76,* 148–151.

SUGGESTED READINGS

Campbell, B., & Morwessel, R. (1998). *Osteoporosis: Time to bone up.* Rosemont, IL: Ruth Jackson Orthopaedic Society.

Glendening, P. N., & Wasserman, M. P. (1998). *Project osteoporosis '98 moving ahead: Launching a community education program.* Annapolis, MD: Department of Health and Mental Hygiene.

Gray, M. A. (1994). Osteoporosis medications: What's your source of information? *Orthopaedic Nursing, 13*(5), 55–58.

Herzberg, M. A. (1997). *Osteoporosis independent study.* Pitman, NJ: National Association of Orthopaedic Nurses.

Hunt, A. H. (1996). The relationship between height change and bone mineral density. *Orthopaedic Nursing, 15*(3), 57–64.

Hunt, A. H. (1998). Metabolic conditions. In A. B. Maher, S. W. Salmond, & T. A. Pellino (Eds.), *Orthopaedic nursing* (2nd ed., pp. 431–479). Philadelphia: Saunders.

Koval, K. J., & Zuckerman, J. D. (1998). Hip. In K. J. Koval & J. D. Zuckerman (Eds.), *Fractures in the elderly* (pp. 175–192). Philadelphia: Lippincott-Raven.

Lane, N. E. (1999). *The osteoporosis book.* New York: Oxford University Press.

Lappe, J. M. (1998). Prevention of hip fractures: A nursing imperative. *Orthopaedic Nursing, 17*(3), 15–24.

Liddel, D. B. (1985). An in-depth look at osteoporosis. *Orthopaedic Nursing, 4*(3), 23–27.

Liscum, B. (1992). Osteoporosis: The silent disease. *Orthopaedic Nursing, 11*(4), 21–25.

National Institute of Arthritis and Musculoskeletal and Skin Diseases, National Institutes of Health. (1986). Osteoporosis: Cause, treatment, prevention. *Orthopaedic Nursing, 5*(6), 29–38.

National Osteoporosis Foundation. (1998). *Physician's guide to prevention and treatment of osteoporosis.* Washington, DC: National Osteoporosis Foundation.

National Osteoporosis Foundation. (1998). *Pocket guide to prevention and treatment of osteoporosis.* Washington, DC: National Osteoporosis Foundation.

Sedlak, C. A., Doheny, M. O., & Jones, S. L. (1998). Osteoporosis prevention in young women. *Orthopaedic Nursing, 17*(3), 53–60.

Tresolini, C. P., Gold, D. T., & Lee, L. S. (Eds.). (1996). *Working with patients to prevent, treat, and manage osteoporosis: A curriculum guide for the health professions.* San Francisco, CA: National Fund for Medical Education.

Appendix

Resources

Calcium Information Center
The New York Hospital Cornell
  Medical Center
515 East 71st Street, Suite 904
New York, NY 10021
212-746-1617

**The International Osteoporosis
  Foundation**
Veronique Forterre, IOF Office
  Manager
71 Cours Albert Thomas
69003 Lyon, France
0033 4 72 914177 Fax 0033 4 72
  369052
http://www.effo.org/

**Hadassah-Women's Zionist
  Organization of America**
National Health Education
  Department
50 West 58th Street
New York, NY 10019
212-303-8139
http://www.hadassah.org/

**National Institute on Aging
  Information Center**
P.O. Box 2577
Gaithersburg, MD 20898-8057
800-222-2225
http://www.nih.gov/nia/

**National Institute of Arthritis
  and Musculoskeletal & Skin
  Disease Information Clearing-
  house**
Box AMS
90 Rockville Pike
Bethesda, MD 20892
301-496-8188
http://www.nih.gov/niams

**National Osteoporosis
  Foundation**
1150 17th Street NW, Suite 500
Washington, DC 20036-4603
202-223-2226 or 800-223-9994
http://www.nof.org nofmail@nof.org

**STRONG WOMEN: Inside and
  Out**
1901 L. Street NW, Suite 300
Washington, DC 20036
202-736-1656 Fax 202-296-3727

North American Menopause Society
c/o Department of OB/GYN
University Hospitals of Cleveland
2074 Abington Road
Cleveland, OH 44106
216-844-3334
http://www.menopause.org/

Office of Disease Prevention & Health Promotion
United States Public Health Service
Washington, DC 20205
202-472-5660
http://www.osophs.dhhs.gov/

Older Women's League
666 Eleventh Street NE, Suite 700
Washington, DC 20001
202-783-6686
http://www.aoa.dhhs.gov/aoa/dir/
   207.html

The Osteoporosis Center
Hospital for Special Surgery
535 East 70th Street
New York, NY 10021
212-606-1588
http://www.hss.edu/

Osteoporosis and Related Bone Disease National Resource Center
1150 17th Street NW, Suite 500
Washington, DC 20036-4603
202-223-0344
http://www.osteo.org

Osteoporosis Society of Canada
33 Laird Drive
Toronto, Ontario MF6 3S9 Canada
416-696-2663
http://www.osteoporosis.ca/

National Women's Health Network
514 10th Street, Suite 400
Washington, DC 20004
202-628-7814
http://www.womenshealthnetwork.org/

Index

Index